Legal Disclaimer

The information contained in this book is not designed to replace or take the place of any form of medicine or professional medical advice. The information in this book has been provided for educational and entertainment purposes only.

All images in this book are licensed and references made to sources of research. The information contained in this book has been compiled from sources deemed reliable, and it is accurate to the best of the Author's knowledge; however, the Author cannot guarantee its accuracy
and validity and cannot be held liable for any errors or omissions. Changes are periodically made to this book. You must consult your doctor or get professional medical advice before using any of the suggested remedies, techniques, or information in this book.

Upon using the information contained in this book, you agree to hold harmless the Author from and against any damages, costs, and expenses, including any legal fees potentially resulting from the application of any of the information provided by this guide. This disclaimer applies to any damages or injury caused by the use and application, whether directly or indirectly, of any advice or information presented, whether for breach of contract, tort, negligence, personal injury, criminal intent, or under any other cause of action.

You agree to accept all risks of using the information presented inside this book. You need to consult a professional medical practitioner to ensure you are both able and healthy enough to participate in this program.

Not for Re-Sale

All rights reserved. All digital products,E-Books, PDF download, resource material, online content and all physical products are subject to copyright protection. Each digital product, E-Book, PDF download and online content is licensed to a single user only. Customers are not allowed to copy, distribute, share and/or transfer the product/s (and/or their associated username/password) they have purchased to any third party or person. Fines of up to $30,000 may apply to person/s found to be infringing our copyright policy.

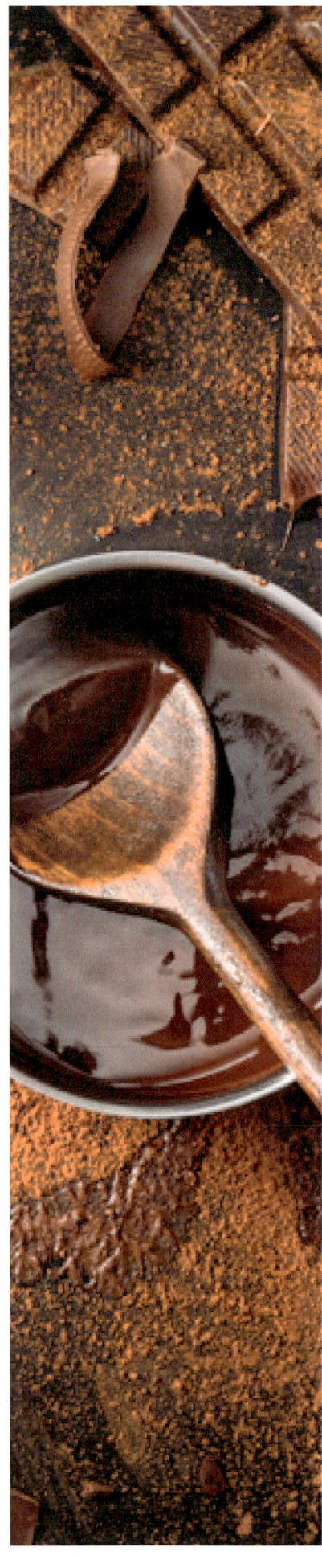

Table of Contents

Introduction — 03
Hi I'm Sarah Jane and this is how my story began.... — 04

Keto Substitutions — 10
Getting in the right mindset — 10
What to expect

Ketosis and the Ketogenic Diet — 11
What is Ketosis? — 12
The Basics of a Ketogenic Diet — 13
Timing — 13
Increasing 'Good Fat' Intake — 14
Balancing out salt or sodium intake — 14
Don't forget the vegetables — 14

Is a Ketogenic Diet Harmful or Dangerous? — 15

How to get started with Keto
Goal setting — 17
Food Choices — 17
Detoxing — 18
7-day meal plan — 18

Transitioning into Keto for Weight Loss — 19
Keep fruits low but eat lots of vegetables. — 20

Fats: The Good, the Bad and the Ugly! — 22
Trans Fats — 22
Saturated Fats — 23
Unsaturated Fats — 23

Recipe Index: — 24

Handy Conversion charts — 97

Glossary — 102
References — 103

Welcome Friends

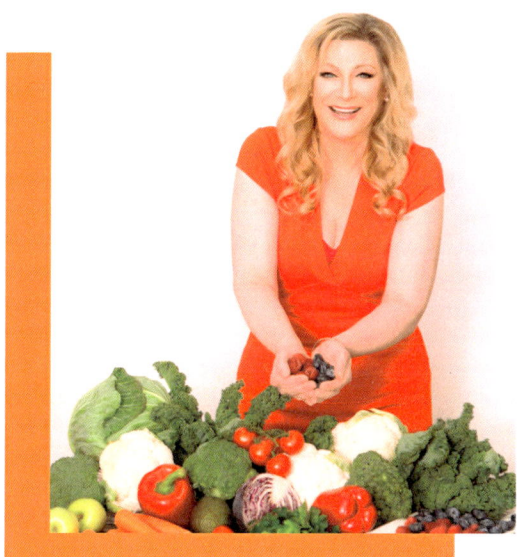

Welcome my lovely friends. It's such a an honour and privilege to welcome you and help you start this journey. It's been literally a lifetime in the making – the journey to be here and then to create this cookbook which I hope brings you what you are seeking.

I have studied and worked for nearly 2 decades as a professional chef. I have designed ,tested and tasted all these recipes to make sure that not only do they work , they also look and taste divine and healthy for you.
The purpose of these recipes is to have that balance between healthy and naughty.
There are 40 recipes in this cookbook. All 40 recipes are made with delicious velvety chocolate*. (sugar free of course) *The chocolate I used in my recipes is called "Well Naturally" sugar free – you may need to find a different version/brand in your country or region.

Every recipe is under 10 grams of net carbohydrates per serve. They are keto friendly (low carbohydrate /high good fats) , sugar free and gluten free.
So, my friends, it is my intention that you enjoy life and your festivities with these recipes whilst at the same time, are also putting good quality ingredients into your body.

Suceess to you always
Sarah Jane

Hi I'm Sarah Jane and this is how my story began....

I have struggled with obesity most of my life. With this struggle, depression and anxiety crept up on me. From the age of 16 I was diagnosed with epilepsy and this resulted in my experiencing grand mal seizures.

After being released from hospital yet again after a traumatic seizure – I reached the lowest point in my life. I had 2 exceptionally large black eyes. My weight had ballooned to an all-time high - I was severely depressed – and I was about to give up on life!

I needed help fast.

They say, **'Sometimes our darkest times are the times that teach us the MOST!'**

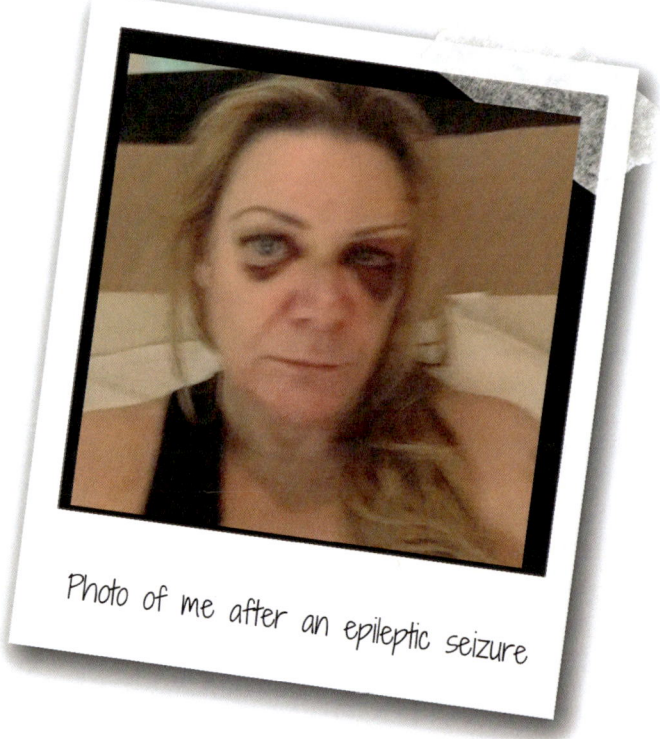

Photo of me after an epileptic seizure

For me – this was very much the TRUTH – this was the moment I turned my life around finally for good!

So, this was the start of my journey....

This is How It All Began.

So then I started to document my journey and created my 1st book to help others:
'I'm Sick of Being Fat!" – How to Lose Weight with Keto

I wrote this book with YOU in mind – because I know there are people in this world – those who are struggling, just like I had, and just want a REAL SOLUTION.

I put everything I learnt into practice and it WORKS!

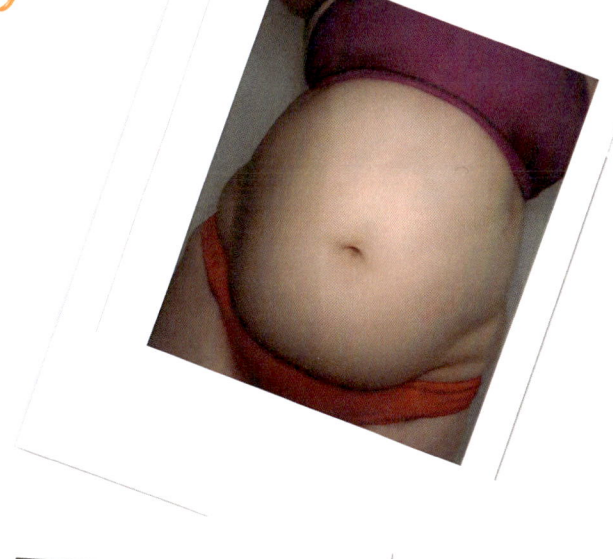

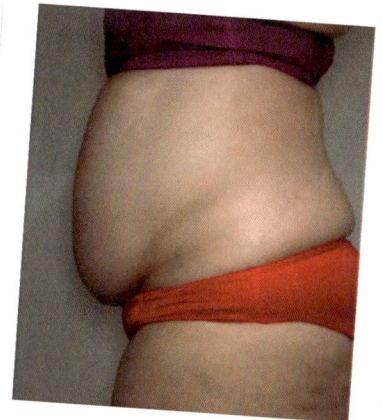

Photos of me at my heavest weight :(

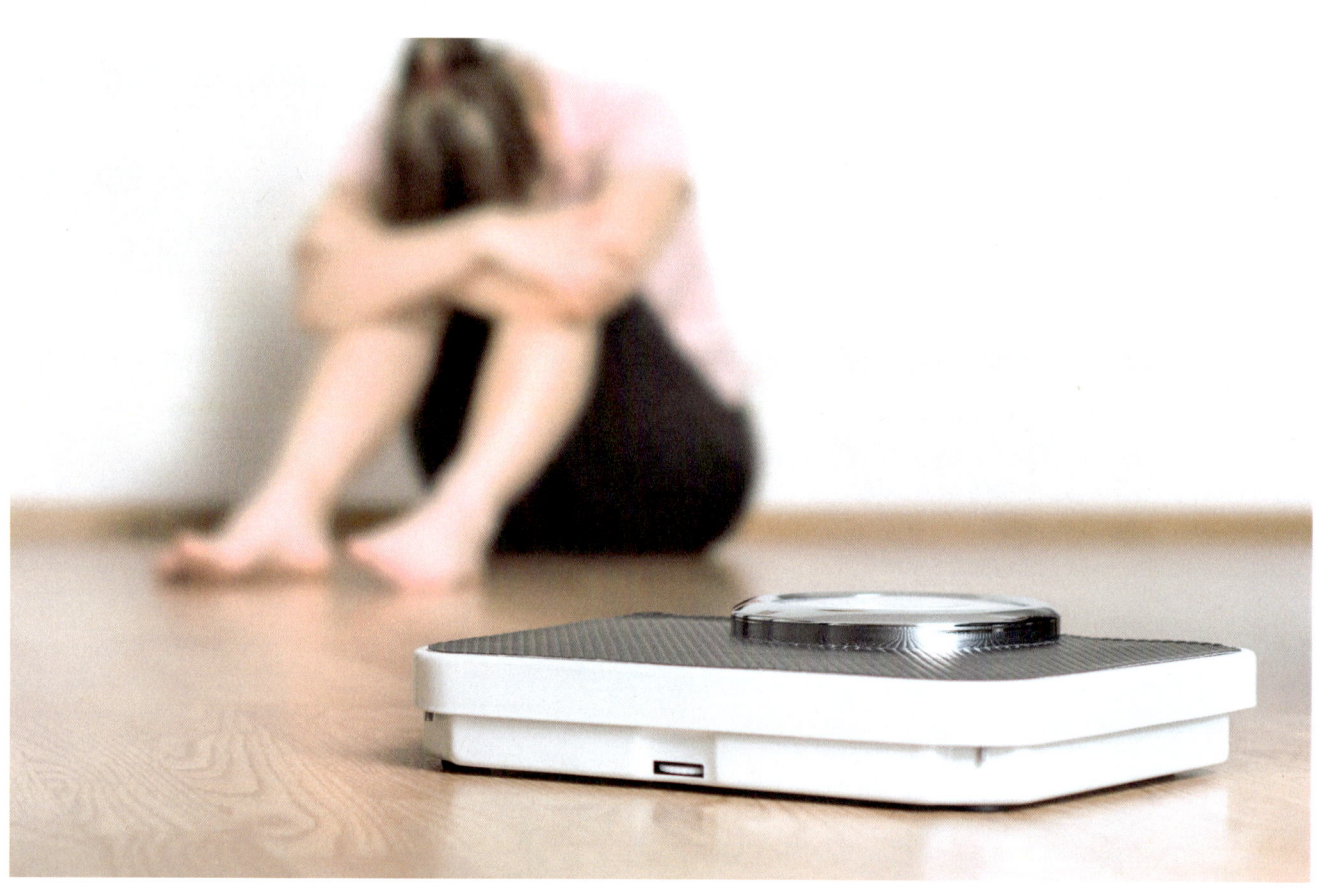

So here is where I decided to change

At the time of this book – I am **down 20 Kg** of body fat – my **waist has shrunk by 12 cm** and I am now happy to say that I am in the 'healthy' measurements.

This is particularly important for visceral fat around the organs – quite dangerous to our health.
I have reduced **dress sizes from 16 to 12** and I still have more to go.

Most exciting for me is that I managed to safely **come off anti-depressants** – I was on them for 6 years and could not get off them and they were NOT helping me.

Best news at the time of writing this book – I have been **seizure free for 2 years!!!!!** *(compared to having 4 seizures in the previous period.)*

Living a Life with a Mission and Purpose

I am living proof that the ketogenic diet is a great solution for many areas including weight loss, epilepsy, depression anxiety, PCOS, Alzheimer's disease, diabetes 2, Parkinson's, and even cancer.

So, my friend – I am excited that you to have decided to ask for help. You are in the right place – I am here to help you and guide you. Let's start your journey together.

If you would like to experience some of your own results then you may like to join our 7 day keto challenge or dive right in to the 30 day program.

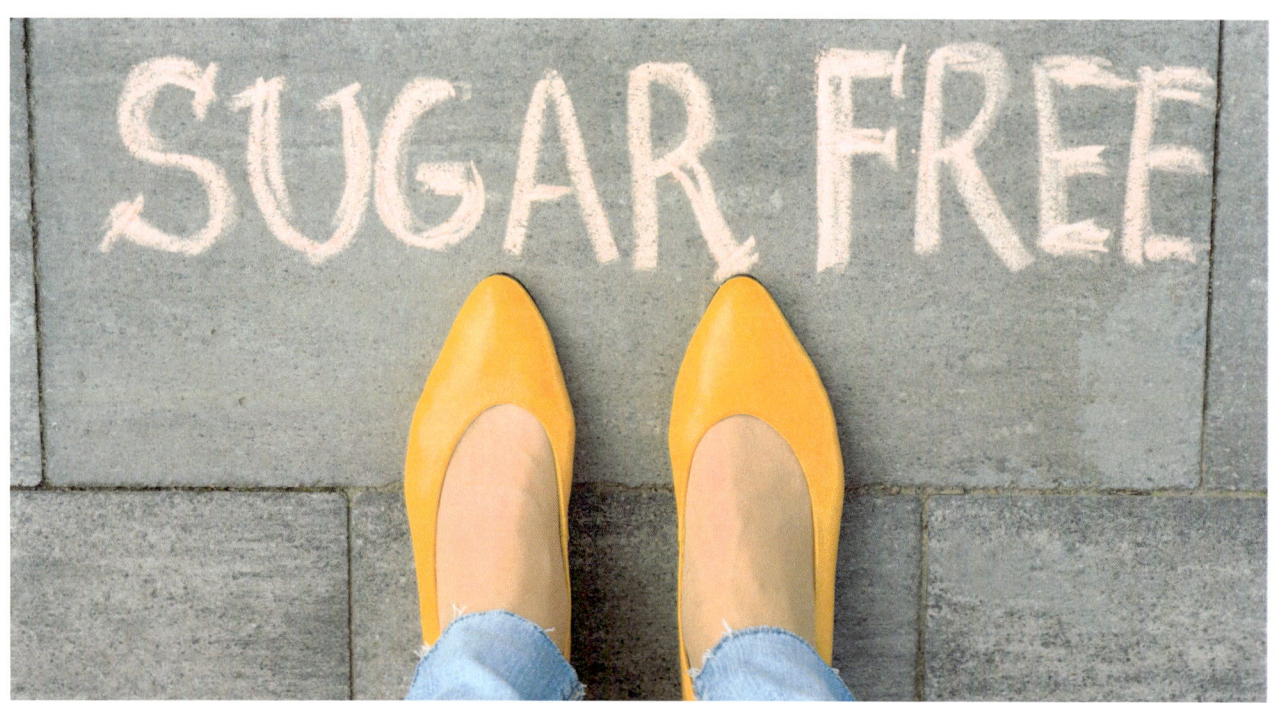

And so She did it too!

Hi, I'm Sarah Jane and that was how my story began.

Fast forward a few years and I am now a **certified Dr Eric Berg health and Keto coach.**

I am studying a **degree in Food and Nutrition** to be a dietitian specialising in the keto diet.

I have authored a book on how to lose weight with the keto diet Released 15 Kg in 12 weeks, Reversed my insulin resistance.

Got myself **free of depression** and anti-depressant medication and reduced the severity and frequency of my epilepsy from 1 every 3 months to **2 years seizure free.**

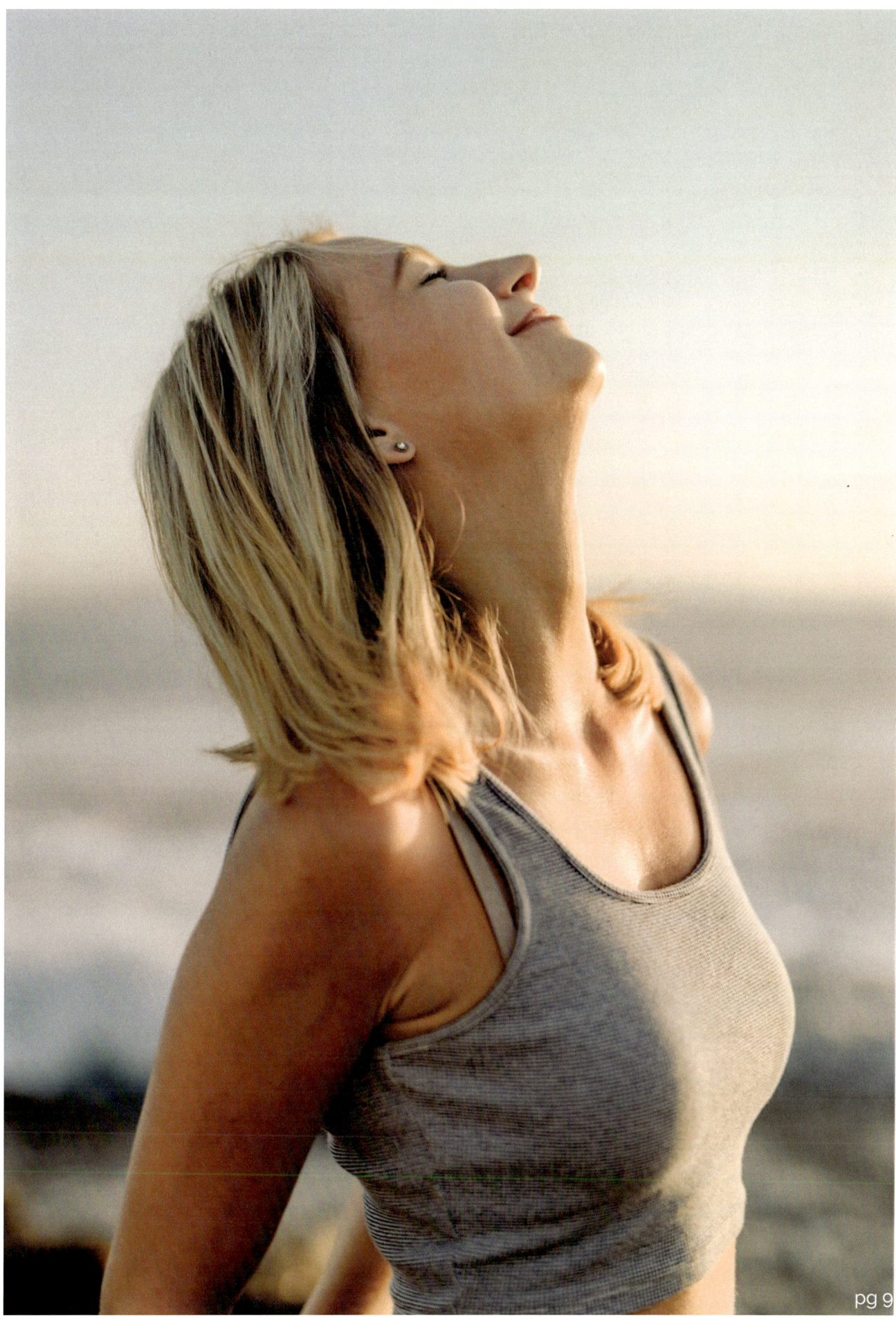

Keto Substitutions

Cooking Oils

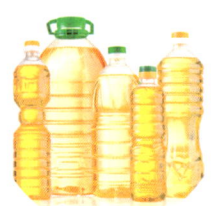

Avoid all of them: vegetable oil, Soybean oil, Corn oil, Canola oil, Sunflower oil, Sesame oil etc. Scientists have hypothesized that too much omega-6 relative to omega-3 may contribute to chronic inflammation

Coconut oil

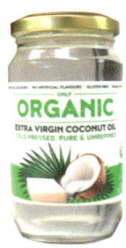

It boosts metabolism and provides a lot of energy. Coconut oil promotes the natural detoxification of the body by metabolizing fats in the liver.

Margarine

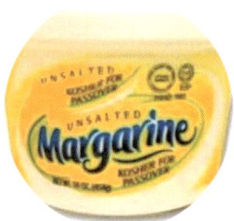

it often contains **trans fat,** which has been associated with an increased risk of heart disease and other chronic health issues

Grass Fed Butter

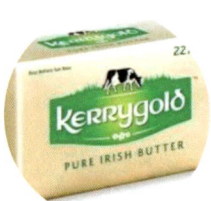

Contains Vitamins A, E and K2. It is also rich in the fatty acids Conjugated Linoleic Acid (CLA) and Butyrate, both of which have powerful health benefits.

Table Salt

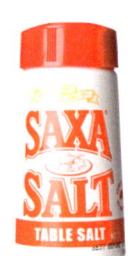

Table salt also goes through a refining process. Anti-caking agents are sometimes added. table salt may have more sodium, but pink Himalayan salt contains more calcium, potassium, magnesium and iron.

Pink Himalayan Rock Salt

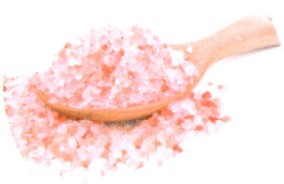

Himalayan salt contains more than 80 minerals and elements, including potassium, iron and calcium

Sugar

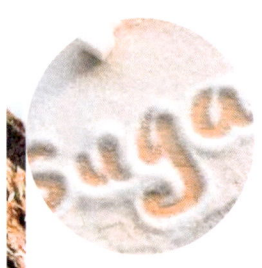

Over time, this can lead to a greater accumulation of fat, which may turn into fatty liver disease, a contributor to diabetes, which raises your risk for heart disease.

Natural Sweetners

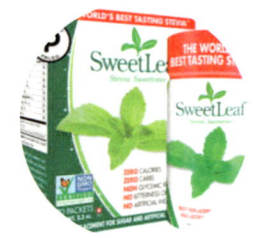

A natural (not an artificial) sweetener with zero calories Stevia may help control Blood sugar and insulin levels

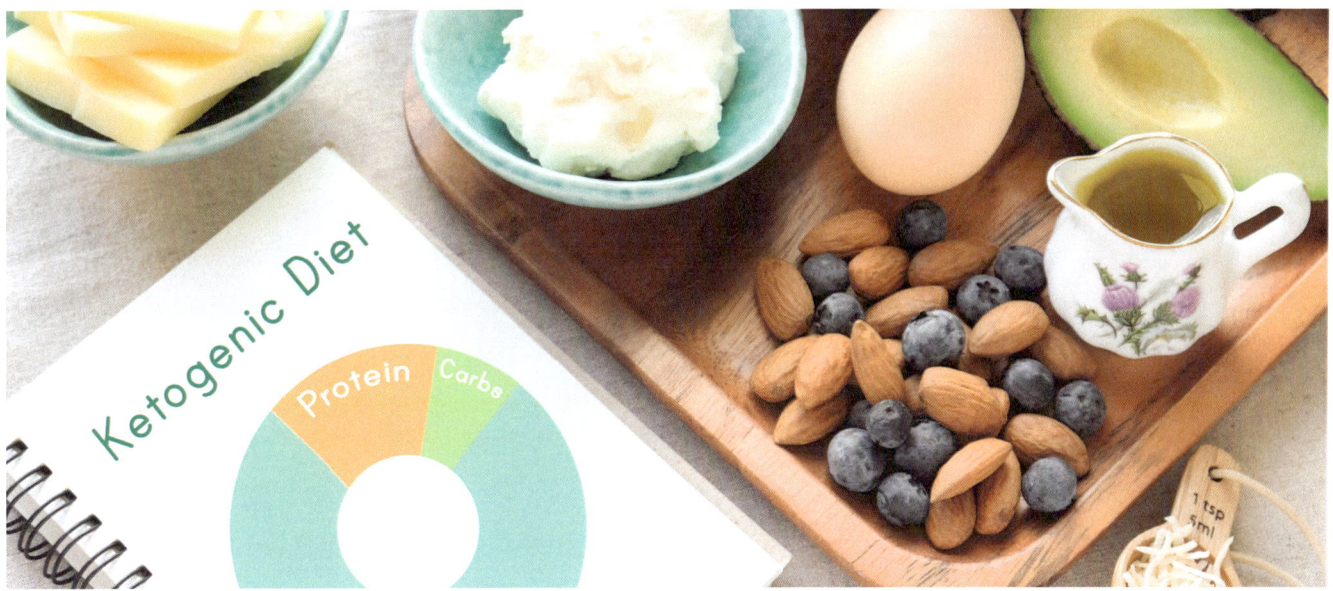

Ketosis and the Ketogenic Diet

What is Ketosis?

In order to help you understand the ketogenic diet and what is involved, you may like to watch my introductory video using the link below. This will help you prepare for what's ahead.

https://www.youtube.com/watch?v=OccowDdcSpk&t=19s

The ketogenic diet is not new and has been in practice since 1920. It involves following a low carbohydrate (10%), moderate protein (20%) and high fat (70%) diet. (A.K.A - LCHF). The ketogenic diet first became popular as a treatment for seizures in children suffering from epilepsy, and the neuro-protective benefits of ketones came to light. As research into the process of ketosis now expands, the list of benefits just continues to grow.

When it comes to adopting a ketogenic diet, focus is usually on consuming less carbs and allowing the body to burn the stored fat in your body as energy. However, a proper ketogenic diet takes so much more into account than just the carbs. It also involves avoiding processed foods that could contain harmful toxins.

The human body is intriguing in many ways, especially when it comes to the production of energy for everyday normal functions.

This energy can come from two (2) sources:

1. the burning of **glucose** /carbohydrates
Or
2. the burning of **fat** (including stored body fat)

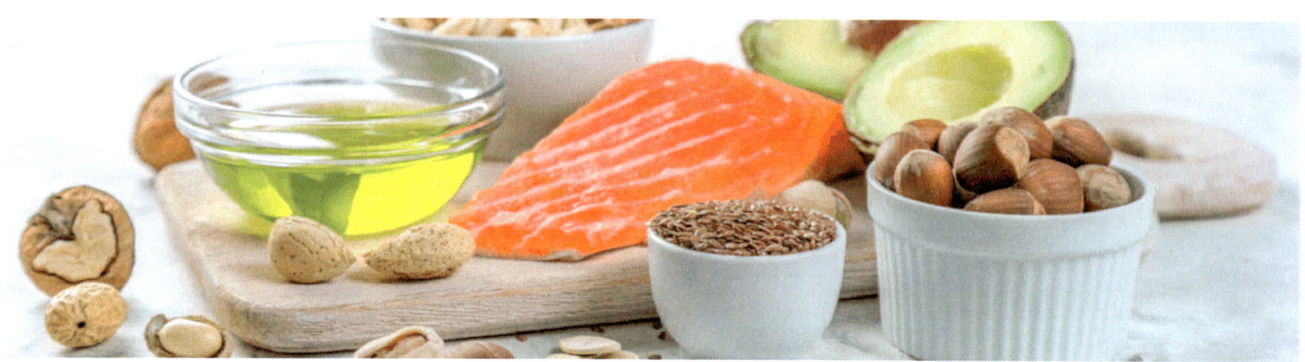

What is Ketosis? (Cont'd)

This is what many refer to as ketosis, a state where the
body obtains its fuel from burning the fat stored in it. The body will often
resort to burning fat when there is little to no glucose in it, making it a
last resort when creating energy for the entire body or a native source of
fuel.

Ideally, if the levels of glucose or the amount of carbs are low enough in the body, it will automatically switch to the breaking down of the fat stored in the body as a source of energy. This is where the benefits of ketosis truly shine through, especially regarding weight loss. When the body
is forced to turn to the stored fat to create energy, excess fat that contributed to weight gain is lost in the process. Ketosis therefore becomes an interesting way to cut down on unnecessary fat in the body, making it a popular weight loss strategy for many people.

On top of cutting down on the body weight, ketosis also results in reduced cravings for food, thanks to a curbed appetite. With a suppressed appetite, it is easy to avoid the unnecessary eating and snacking that is often the cause of excess weight gain. There are so many more benefits that come with ketosis which will come further in this book, but on top of the main benefits that are weight loss and improved body composition, the rest are welcome bonuses.excellence she inquietude contrasted.

The Basics of a Ketogenic Diet

The main purpose of a ketogenic diet is to help your body get used to processing fats for energy. Carbohydrates in the form of starchy carbs/grains are therefore to be avoided at all costs. Most grains such as wheat, rye, quinoa, bread, rice, cakes, cookies, crackers, biscuits and various others are to be avoided. Sugars and sweets are notorious for their high calorie contents and should also be put away. It is also worth noting that most high calorie foods come from processed food, and should also be avoided at all costs

Timing

A ketogenic can often be utilized with 'intermittent fasting' for far more effective results. All the meals that are to be consumed for the day for an individual following a ketogenic diet should be done so within a 6-hour window. This prevents overeating and allows the body more time to focus on burning body fat for energy. It is important that all eating be done a minimum of 3 hours before going to bed, so as not to interfere with human growth hormone production that occurs when we sleep, stalling weight loss altogether. Any eating outside of this time frame should be limited to drinking water or healthy tea, which is fine. Sleep is also an important part of the equation, with 8 hours being the ideal resting time.

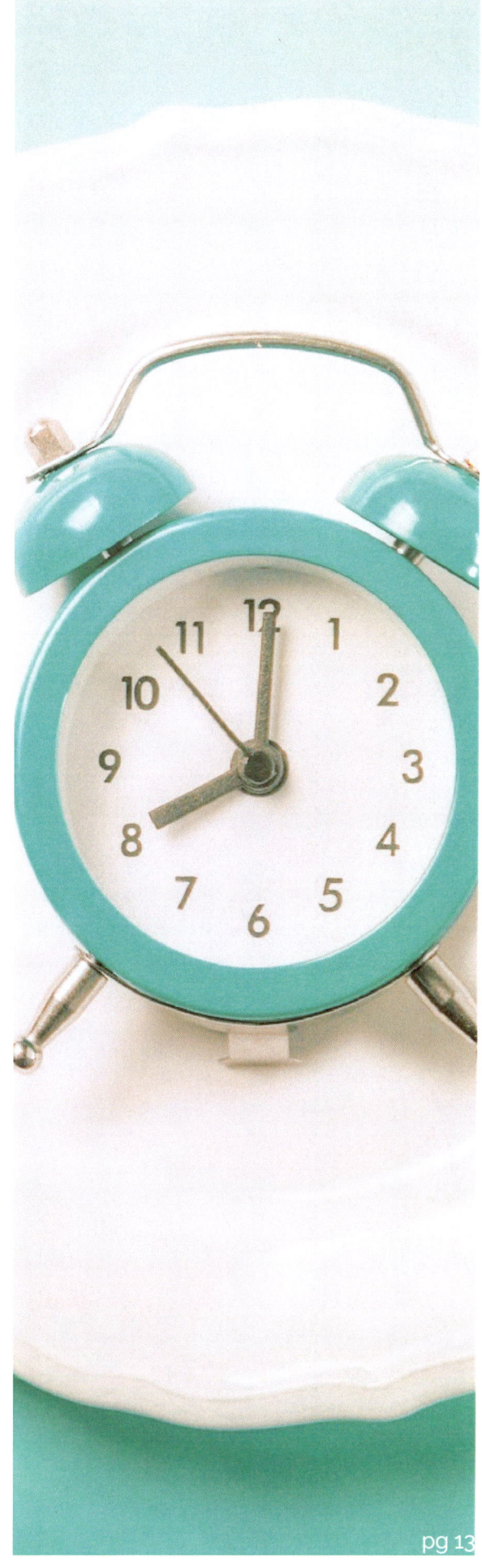

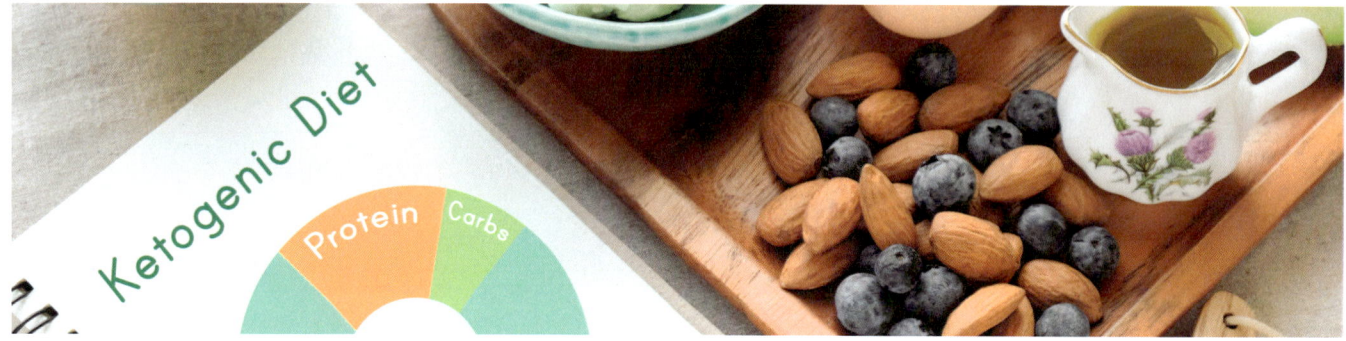

Increasing 'Good Fat' Intake

At a glance, this may sound counterintuitive since you are trying to lose weight by burning fat in the first place. However, a healthy ketogenic diet should also help your body adapt to breaking down fats to produce energy. Since the principal source of energy for your body is fat, it is important to focus on eating foods rich in fat. The kind of fat also matters, as unhealthy fats are counterproductive towards the weight loss goal. Some of the ideal recommended foods include avocados for the mono-saturated fat and omega 3 from seafood and the saturated fats that come from butter and coconut oil.

Balancing out salt or sodium intake

When the body is more focused on carbs as a source of energy, a lot of sodium is often released into the body. When the diet shifts to one focusing more on fats instead, the salt content in the body reduces drastically.

It is therefore important to incorporate foods that add a bit of sodium to the system to balance out the expected deficiency. These include carrots, celery and meat. Also ensure that you always use Pink Himalayan salt. This salt has been found to contain up to 80 different essential minerals that your body need. So contrary to beliefs about salt, this type of salt – not the processed table salt variety is good for your body.

Don't forget the vegetables

Most diets that contribute to weight loss often have the added benefit of also improving the overall body health. This principle also rings true for a ketogenic diet. Non-starchy vegetables like spinach, lettuce, chives, asparagus and cucumbers come highly recommended for their vitamin value.

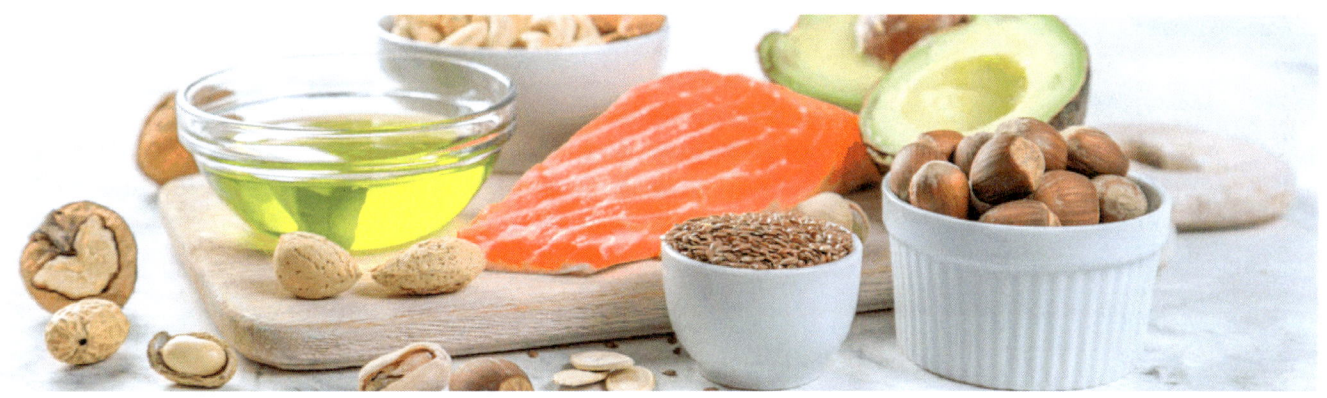

Is a Ketogenic Diet Harmful or Dangerous?

There is a lot of misinformation, myths and general 'un-truths' out there on the internet and the public domain about the keto diet. Many people confuse the term 'ketosis' with the far dangerous state of 'Keto-acidosis'. These are two very different conditions. Keto-acidosis is found in Type 1 diabetics that have extremely dangerous levels of low glucose resulting in this state. Ketosis on the other hand is a very natural process of unlocking fats – either in the form of fats we eat or body fats, to fuel the body for metabolic energy. Keto-acidosis therefore would only occur if you were a type 1 diabetic or if you had literally starved for well over a month.

Additionally, the data and actual studies that are formulated are based on incorrect data collated from false criteria from the onset. Often when these clinical studies were initiated they were performed on rodents, mice and rats.

The actual "high fat' diet they were fed for the studies was NOT actually a traditional ketogenic diet. Instead what the rodents were fed was a HIGH FAT/HIGH CARB diet – which is NOT a ketogenic diet and YES that would be dangerous. As already explained a keto diet is LOW CARB/HIGH FAT. Specifically, the results from these clinical studies demonstrate the actual macro breakdown to:

- 24% carbs,
- 21% protein
- And 50% fats.

Comparatively a traditional keto diet is:

- 5-10% carbs
- 20 % protein
- And 70-75% fats.

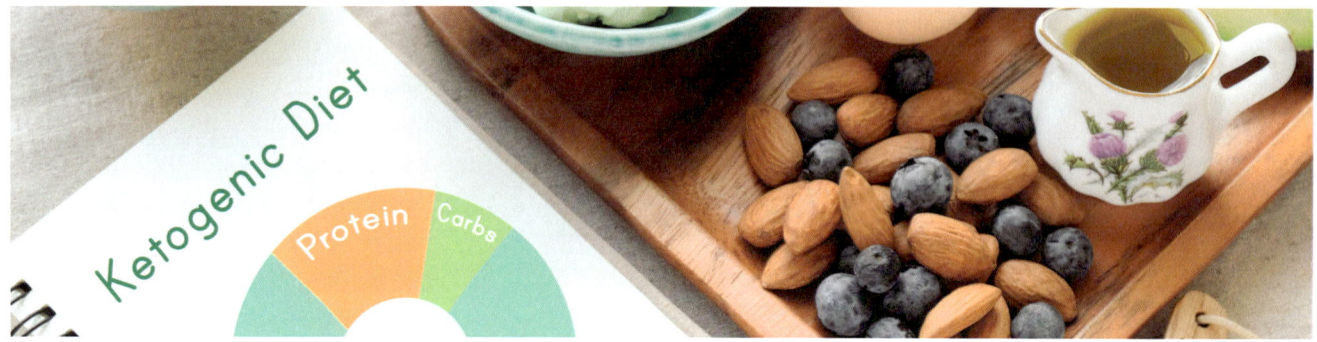

Is a Ketogenic Diet Harmful or Dangerous? (Cont'd)

Going further into detail on exactly what type's /categories as well as quality of fats the rodent consumed during the experiment also sheds further light on the myths surrounding keto diets.
The QUALITY of the fats they were fed were indeed dangerous. In fact, 30% of the fat intake was of a 'Trans Fat' category, which as we have already explained in this book thus far, is, indeed highly dangerous and should be AVOIDED. The Ketogenic diet does NOT encourage anyone to consume these in any levels – These are present in processed and manufactured foods.
Next 28% was consumed from the 'saturated fat 'category – which is the animal fats. A ketogenic diet does allow only a moderate-to- low consumption of these. Finally, the Unsaturated fats category – the plant-based fats - including Polyunsaturated and Mono-Unsaturated fats) this category showed the rodents eating LEAST OF– whereas a traditional ketogenic diet favours the unsaturated fats to be MOST consumed

So, you can see the actual studies themselves were incorrectly set up and therefore the result of which do not actually test a ketogenic diet – what these studies do show Is that a diet that is based on manufactured foods, poor quality hydrogenated oils, and high carb intake combined all leads to a dangerous result.

This is true!

So instead –when someone does say that a keto diet' is dangerous - ask the source of the clinical study.

I have attached the link to the actual data, so you can check it out yourself.

http://diabetes.diabetesjournals.org/content/diabetes/suppl/2009/08/18/db08-1261.DC1/db08-1261_Online_appendix.pdf

How to get started with Keto

The main reason why we gain and have difficulty losing fat, particularly in those stubborn areas, is related to very specific hormones. These hormones have an effect on whether we hold onto fat or whether we burn fat. These are all run by the endocrine system in our body.

The main hormonal '*culprits*' for weight issues are:

- Insulin
- Insulin resistance
- Cortisol
- Estrogen

Mindset

Mindset is a big part of weight loss- How we think and what we say to ourselves in our mind has a huge effect on how we feel about ourselves and the actions we take or don't take in life that consequently give us the results we have now.

Goal setting

It is important to clearly state what you want to achieve. Choose your 'WHY'. Losing weight is NOT easy – even if so many weight loss programs will tell you it is – it's hard work – so you
need to have the right MINDSET and know why you are doing this. I imagine it will be because of the love of your children, family and ultimately yourself and for general health and well-being.

Food Choices

Choosing the right types of foods particularly those that are natural fat burners as well as having additional health benefits. By merely substituting some ingredients you currently eat, with these, you will be making small but consistent steps forward to your end goal.

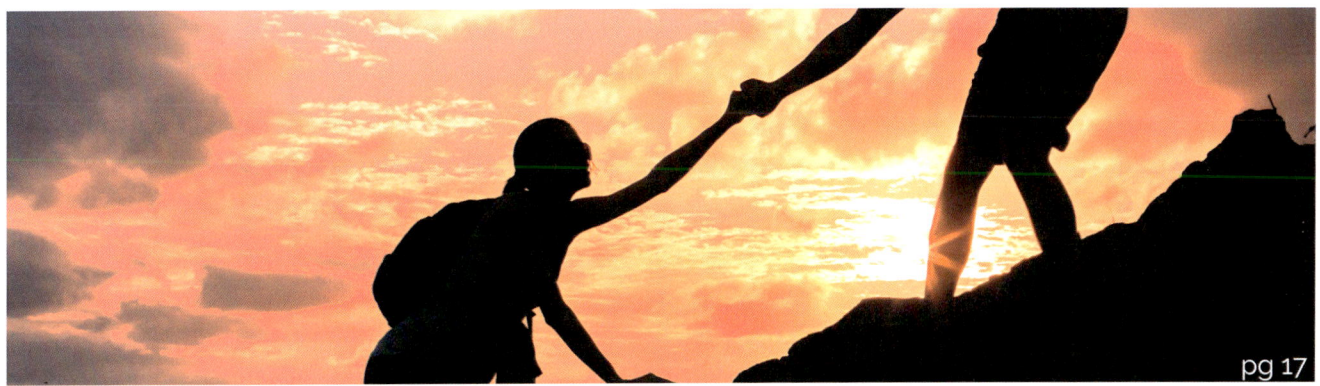

How to get started with Keto

Detoxing
You will need to detox away from all high sugar, processed and manufactured foods. Start looking for REAL foods instead of something that comes out of a box from a factory. Get back to basics. Strip away all the inflammatory food. Start to 'listen' to your body. If something gives you pain, indigestion, excessive wind, acne, etc., it means it's inflammatory to your body. Listen to your body's signs and either eliminate those foods or substitute for something healthier.

7-day meal plan
If you would additional meal planning there is a free e-book at ketotrans4mations.com with a "*7 day keto Kickstarter*". Includes meal plan, shopping list, recipes. This is a low calorie standard meal plan that will help you to lose weight. The average in the first 7 days 24 hour is 2Kg however results vary from person to person.

We provided you with an introduction to the science behind a ketogenic diet, what is involved, what are the myths and what are the multiple benefits of following such a diet. Overall, the main aim is to get you healthy, and once your body is healthy and all your hormones are balanced and working properly, you WILL naturally lose the body fat. The weight is just a symptom that your body is not healthy.

So, in this next chapter, let me tell you how to transition into a keto diet which will OPTIMISE your fat loss and literally melt that fat away that you have been trying so hard to get rid of.

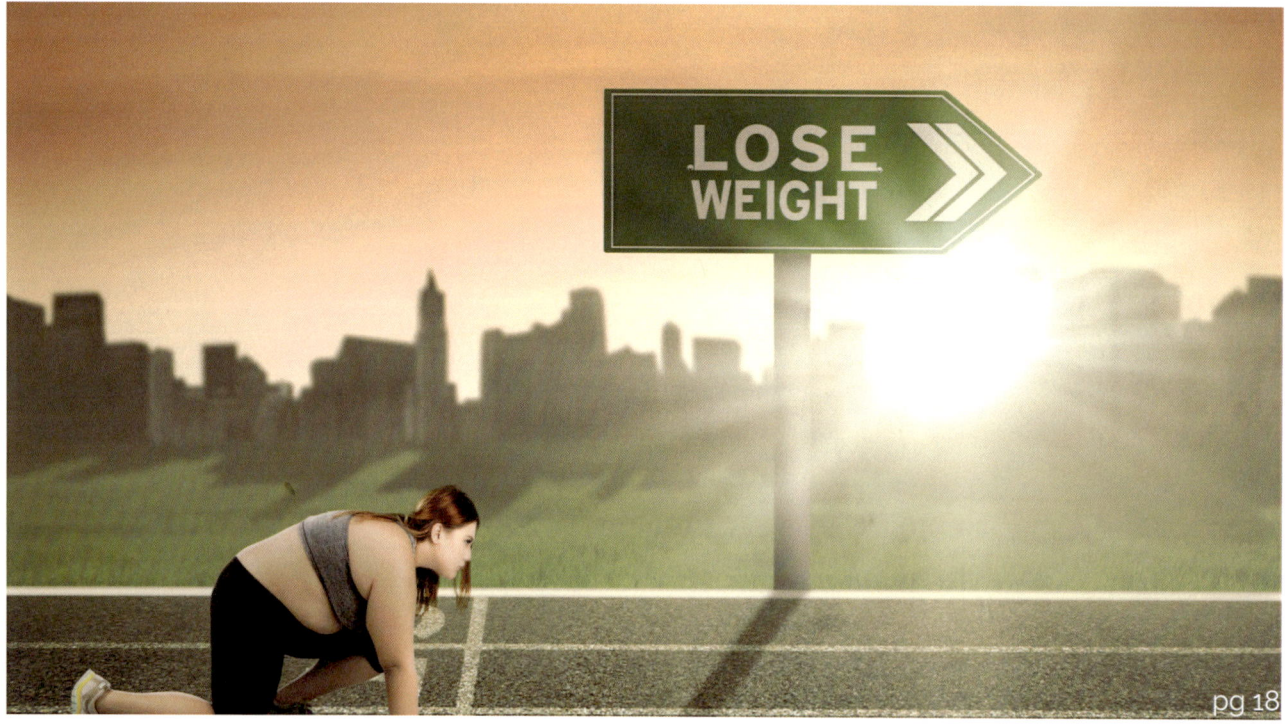

Transitioning into Keto for Weight Loss

As we have covered previously, the body traditionally uses glucose (or carbohydrates) as its main source of energy. However, there is another source which the body can use and that is through fats. Now, fats can come in 2 forms, either:

1. Fats that we eat
2. Or stored body fats

It is through the liver and mitochondria that ketone bodies will break down fats so that it can be used as an alternative source of metabolic energy to fuel its needs.

Now, up until now – reading this book, you have always been told that the only way to burn fat and lose weight is to cut calories and go into a calorie deficit. – Basically, starving yourself of your body's nutritional needs.

Now, don't get me wrong, being in a calorie deficit is helpful short term and in itself is a metabolic state of endogenous ketosis– however, it's the nutrients, the macro-components and the QUALITY that makes up those calories that we are going to focus on with keto.

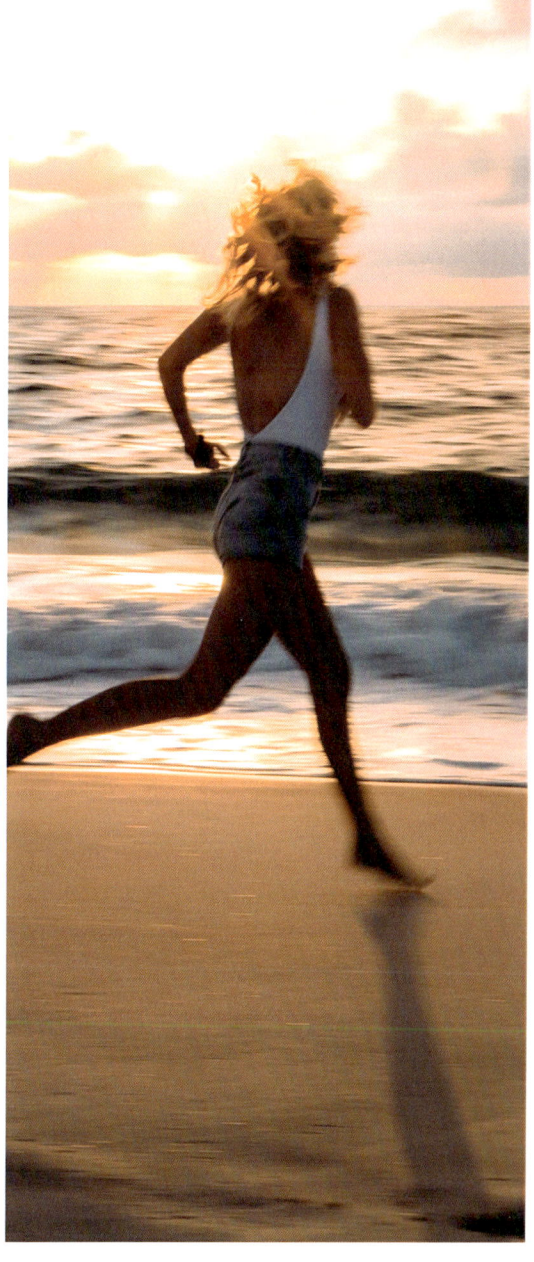

Transitioning into Keto for Weight Loss (Cont'd)

First step you would need to take when you first began our 7 day keto challenge would have been a carb detox or a 24 hour fast preferably. This is an important stage as the body cannot use 2 different types of fuel at the same time. It will either favour one or the other. So, we need to shift over and transition away from a diet that is high in carbohydrates. Now, for clarity, carbohydrates include:

- Complex carbohydrates
- Simple Carbohydrates

Many of us know the complex carbohydrates
- our breads, pastas, rice, oats, wheat, grains, etc.

Simple carbohydrates are fruits and vegetables and the more obvious processed sugars. So, you need to be conscious of the simple carbohydrates you are eating as well as those 'hidden' carbs that are found in products, sauces, dressings, etc. Even dairy can be high in carbohydrates particularly yoghurts, so watch these! Many people often discover they are intolerant of dairy (lactose) and find it is a cause of inflammation.

Keep fruits low but eat lots of vegetables.

You will be getting all your macro carbohydrates from the vegetables and fruits as well as your micro-nutrients -all the essential vitamins and minerals that your body needs. So, eat as much leafy green non-starchy vegetables as you like. Limit fruit and AVOID starchy carbs.

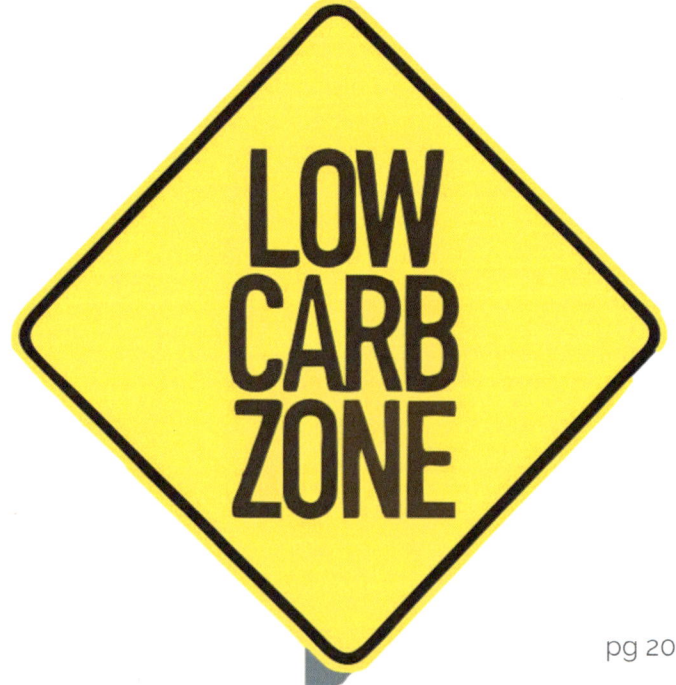

Transitioning into Keto for Weight Loss (Cont'd)

When you move into keto, your macro breakdown is going to look like this:

10% Carbohydrates
20% Protein
70% Fats

Now, most people usually freak out when they initially hear the high fat component. So please, before you do that, give yourself a chance to understand the process through this book and my videos - how the body works and why this is such an effective way of losing weight as well as fuelling the body with everything it needs.

I admit it does seem counter intuitive, as it did for me, that by eating fat you can lose weight. A lot of it comes down to the way we have always been educated on food and nutrition. Even from school age with the food pyramid telling us to eat breads and cereals the 'most ',and fats the 'least'.

Yet millions of people around the world are suffering from obesity and it's growing bigger into epidemic proportions. Weight related diseases are at an all-time high that could be prevented and indeed reversed with proper health and nutrition.

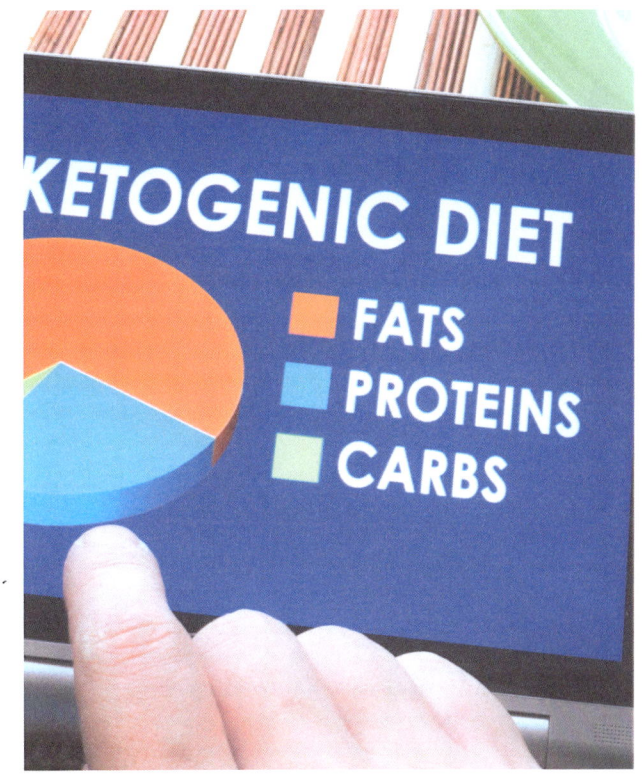

To help you understand a little more about why the keto diet is so effective, I am going to explain more about what fats do in the body, why you need them, which ones to eat, and which to avoid:

Along with protein, fats have an essential function in the body.

- Fats give you energy.
- Keep your body warm.
- They build your cells.
- Protect your organs.
- Help your body absorb essential vitamins and minerals from your food.
- And they produce the hormones that your body needs to work properly.

Fats: The Good, the Bad and the Ugly!

Not all fat are created equal.
Getting down to basics, there are 3 separate categories when it comes to dietary fats.

1. Trans-fats (Ugly) Avoid
2. Saturated fats (bad) Moderate
3. Unsaturated fats (Good) Most

The difference between these three (3) types of fats lies in their chemical composition.
All fats are made up of carbon atoms that are linked or bonded to a hydrogen atom.

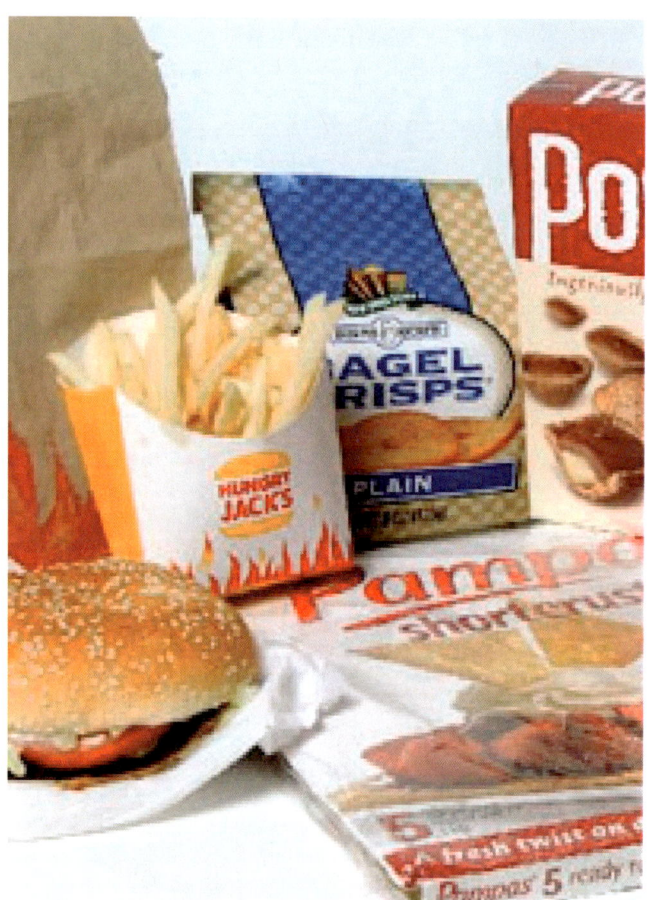

Trans Fats

Trans Fats are the manufactured fats that have gone through a process called 'hydrogenation'.

You'll probably see these listed on your ingredients labelled as
'partly -hydrogenated oils' to disguise the fact that these are actually trans fats.

Trans fats are created to make foods:

· Last longer on the shelf/supermarket
· Improve the taste
· Improve the texture

You'll find trans-fat in cakes, pies, cookies, biscuits, crackers, margarine, etc. All those yummy things – *right*!

But whilst Trans Fats may taste good – they are NOT good for you!!

AVOID Trans Fats at all costs!

Saturated Fats

Saturated fats are where the carbon atoms are completely covered with a hydrogen atom or *"saturated"*, and this is also what makes them solid at room temperature. Saturated fats are basically your **animal fats** like cheese, butter, yoghurt, cream, eggs and coconut oil, feel free to eat these in **MODERATION**.

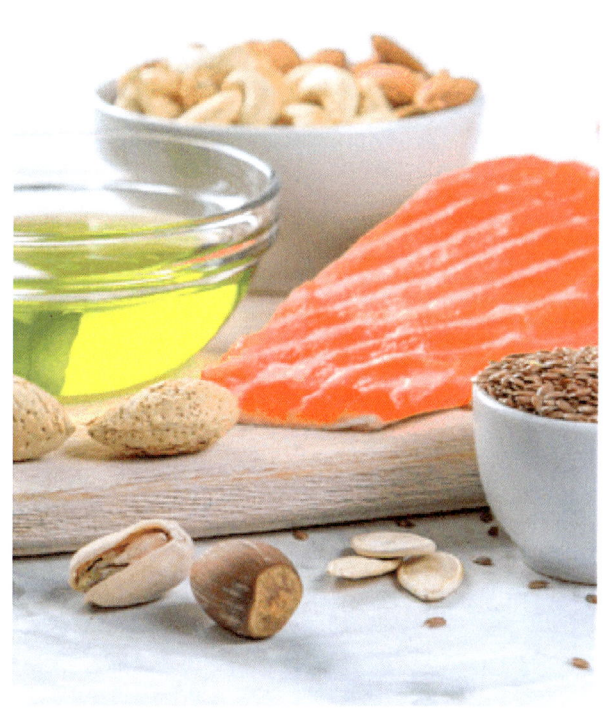

Unsaturated Fats

Unsaturated fats have fewer carbon atoms that are bonded and hence liquid at room temperature.

These are the Fats that I want you to the <u>**EAT MOST OF.**</u>

These are mainly plant-based fats. These are broken down into 2 more types:

1. Monounsaturated
2. Polyunsaturated

Your heart and your brain absolutely LOVE these Unsaturated fats.

Monounsaturated Fats

Mono' meaning one, has one carbon bond attached. These are your avocados, olive oils, peanut oils, nuts: almonds, hazelnuts and macadamias.

Polyunsaturated Fats

'Poly' – meaning '*many*' carbon bonds attached. These are your 'Essential Fatty Acids'. (EFA)

Flaxseeds, walnuts, leafy green vegetables, fatty fish, salmon tuna, mackerel, and sardines.

These are going to give you your Omega 3 and Omega 6s.

Recipe Index:
40 All chocolate, no sugar, low-carb, keto friendly recipes

Truffles

Valencia Orange Choc Truffles	p. 25
Chocolate & Macadamia Truffles	p. 26
Chocolate Peanut Butter Truffles	p. 27
Choc Coconut Bites	p. 28
Chocolate Coated Meringues	p. 29

Slices

Chocolate & Walnut Slice	p. 30
Chocolate Peanut Slice	p. 31
Chocolate Caramel Slice	p. 32
Chocolate Nutty Bars	p. 34

Brownies/muffins/friands/donuts

Double Chocolate Brownies	p. 36
My 'Turkish Delight'	p. 37
Chocolate Swirl Muffins	p. 39
Chocolate- Zucchini Muffins	p. 41
White Chocolate Friands	p. 43
Mmmm!....Donuts	p. 45
Chocolate Waffles	p. 45

Biscuits

Chocolate Chip Cookies	p. 47
'Choc-Mint Slices'	p. 50
Viennese Fingers	p. 52

Snacks
(*names changed to protect the innocent)

Éclairs	p. 53
Pitch Your 'Wagon Wheels'	p. 55
'Venus' Bars (Not from' Mars')	p. 57
White Chocolate – Sugar Free	p. 60
'Snackers' Bar	p. 61
Chocolate Hazelnut Spread	p. 63
A.k.a 'Nutella'	p. 65
Pop your 'Cherry Ripe' Bars	
Mutiny on the 'Bounty' Bars	p. 67
Twax' Bars	p. 69
	p. 71

Desserts

Chocolate Mousse	p. 73
No-Sugar Chocolate Ice Cream	p. 74
Chocolate Soufflé	p. 75
Chocolate Panna Cotta	p. 78
Steamed Chocolate Orange Pudding	p. 80
with Chocolate Custard	p. 81
Dairy Free -Chocolate Mousse	p. 82
Chocolate Truffle Crème Brule.	p. 83

Cakes

Baked Chocolate Cheesecake	p. 84
Sacher Torte	p. 87
Ganache Tart with Crunchy	p. 89
Macadamia, Pistachio and	p. 91
Coconut Topping	
Tiramisu Swiss Roll	p. 91
Black Forrest Gateau	p. 94

Valencia Orange Choc Truffles

These delectable truffles are sure to keep you coming back for more. With an orange aroma and cacao nib crunch, your senses will be delighted.

Yield: Makes approx. 12 Truffles

Ingredients

135g Sugar free dark chocolate
¼ tsp orange oil or essence
6 tsps. Coconut cream
2 tsps. Coconut oil
2 tsps. Cacao Nibs

Coating

½ cup Cacao Powder

DIRECTIONS

1: Melt the chocolate in a heat proof container in the microwave for approximately 1 min, stirring with a metal spoon until smooth.

2: Once melted, add the coconut cream and cacao nibs.

3: Spread the mix onto a large, flat tray lined with baking paper and place in the freezer until it just starts to firm (approx. 3-5 minutes).

4: Once the mix has started to firm and is dough-like to touch, wet your hands in cold water and pick up teaspoon-size pieces of the mix.

5: Roll the mix into balls in the palm of your hands and then dust with the cacao powder for coating.

6: Place back onto the lined tray and refrigerate until firm.

7: Remove from the fridge 10 minutes before serving.

Nutrition Facts

Amount per 1 serving (0.7 oz) 19 g
Calories 28   From Fat 20
% Daily Value*
Total Fat 2.4g — 4%
Saturated Fat 1.8g — 9%
Trans Fat 0g
Cholesterol 0mg — 0%
Sodium 43mg — 2%
Total Carbohydrates 4g — 1%
Dietary Fiber 2g — 7%
Sugars 0g
Protein 1g — 2%
Vitamin A 0% • Vitamin C 0%
Calcium 1% • Iron 5%
* Percent Daily Values are based on 2000 calorie diet. Your Daily Values may be higher or lower depending on your calorie needs.
HappyForks.com

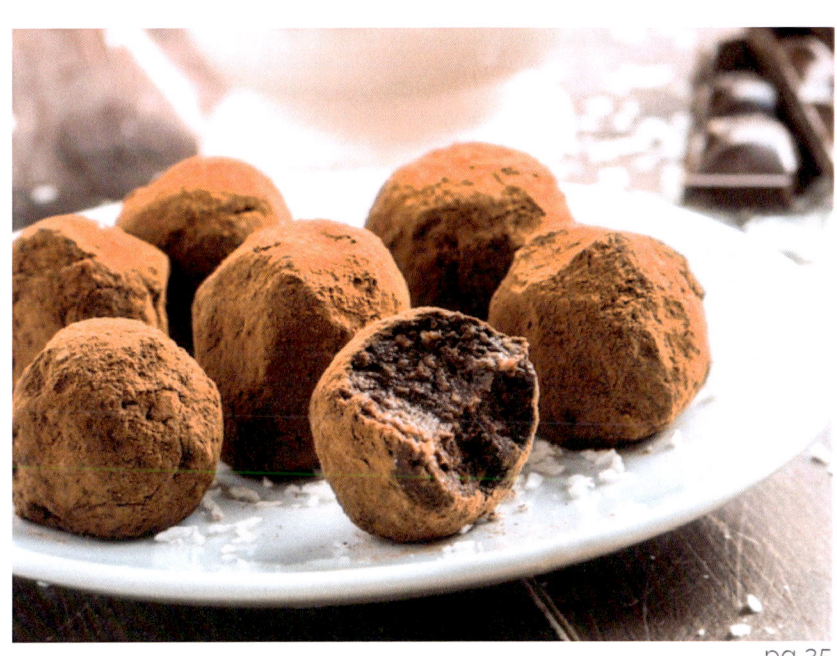

Chocolate & Macadamia Truffles

These chocolate and macadamia truffles are the perfect bite-sized treats to keep to yourself or share with loved ones. You're bound to go 'nuts' over these!

Serves 16 truffles

Ingredients

135g Sugar free dark chocolate

2 tsps. Coconut oil

6 tsps. Coconut cream

Pinch Of salt

6 Tbsp Crushed macadamias

Coating

½ cup Crushed macadamias

DIRECTIONS

1: Melt the chocolate in a heat proof container in the microwave for approximately 1 min, stirring with a metal spoon until smooth.

2: Once it has melted, add the coconut cream, macadamias and salt.

3: Spread the mix onto a large, flat plate lined with baking paper and place in the freezer until it just starts to firm (approx. 3-5 minutes).

4: Once the mix has started to firm and is dough-like to touch, wet your hands in cold water and pick up teaspoon-size pieces of the mix.

5: Roll the mix into balls and then into the crushed macadamias for coating.

6; Place onto a tray lined with baking paper andrefrigerate until firm.

7: Remove from the fridge 10 minutes before serving.

Nutrition Facts

Amount per 1 serving (0.7 oz) 19 g

Calories 75 — From Fat 65

% Daily Value*

- Total Fat 7.7g — 12%
- Saturated Fat 2.1g — 11%
- Trans Fat 0g
- Cholesterol 0mg — 0%
- Sodium 39mg — 2%
- Total Carbohydrates 2g — 1%
- Dietary Fiber 1g — 4%
- Sugars 0g
- Protein 1g — 2%
- Vitamin A 0% • Vitamin C 0%
- Calcium 1% • Iron 3%

* Percent Daily Values are based on 2000 calorie diet. Your Daily Values may be higher or lower depending on your calorie needs.

HappyForks.com

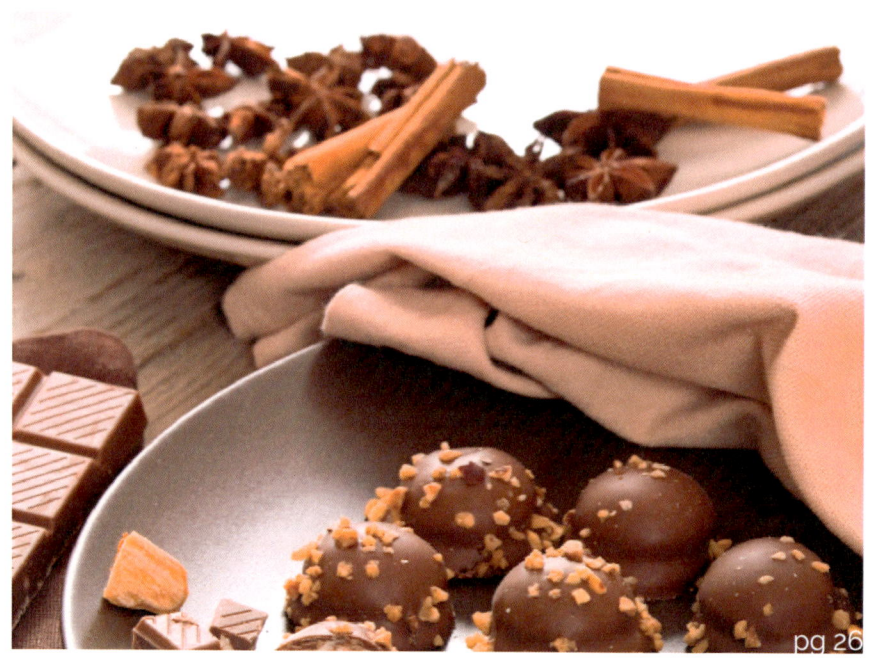

Chocolate Peanut Butter Truffles

The classic combination of chocolate and peanut butter, these little truffles are reminiscent of a 'REESE'S Peanut Butter Cup'. They are the perfect companion for movies, sports and parties.

Yield: Makes Approx.20

Ingredients

Peanut Butter Caramel

8-10 Medjool dates
(*Soft, pitted*)

1 cup Peanut butter
(*Smooth, natural*)

⅓ cup Coconut flour

1 Tbsp Chia seeds (optional)

A pinch Pink Himalayan salt

Chocolate Coating:

200g Sugar free dark chocolate

1 tsps. Coconut oil

DIRECTIONS

1: Process the pitted dates in a food processor until they form a sticky paste.

2: Add the peanut butter, chia seeds and salt, followed by the coconut flour, and process until the mixture is smooth and well combined. The mixture will be slightly sticky.

3: Transfer the mixture to a bowl and freeze, uncovered, for about 10 minutes (this will make it easier to shape).

4: Using a teaspoon, scoop the chilled mixture and shape into small balls using the palms of your hands, then place on a lined tray and place back in the freezer for approx. 10 minutes, until firm.

5: Melt the sugar free dark chocolate and add the coconut oil, stirring until smooth and glossy. Allow to cool slightly before coating.

6: Remove balls from the freezer and coat each one with the melted chocolate before placing onto the lined tray.

7: Chill in the refrigerator for half an hour, or until the chocolate coating is set.

Nutrition Facts

Amount per
1 serving (1.4 oz) — 40 g

Calories 114	From Fat 46
	% Daily Value*
Total Fat 5.5g	8%
Saturated Fat 1.1g	6%
Trans Fat 0g	
Cholesterol 0mg	0%
Sodium 124mg	5%
Total Carbohydrates 15g	5%
Dietary Fiber 2g	8%
Sugars 9g	
Protein 4g	9%
Vitamin A 0% • Vitamin C	0%
Calcium 2% • Iron	4%

* Percent Daily Values are based on 2000 calorie diet. Your Daily Values may be higher or lower depending on your calorie needs.

HappyForks.com

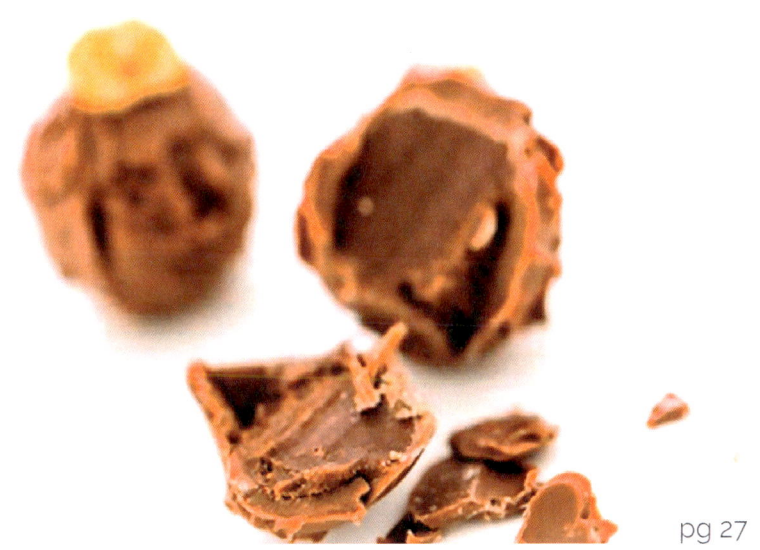

Choc Coconut Bites

Yield: Makes Approx. 15 bites

Ingredients

1 cup Shredded coconut

1½ cups Desiccated coconut

2 Tbsp Sugar-free fibre syrup (ie Sukrin)

½ tsps. Vanilla extract

2 Tbsp Coconut oil

¼ cup Coconut milk

150g Sugar-free dark chocolate

DIRECTIONS

1: Put everything except the chocolate into a food processor and blitz for 30 seconds or until combined.

2: Remove the blade, scrape down the sides and ensure it's mixed well.

3: Roll the coconut mixture into small balls, place onto a tray lined with baking paper and transfer to the freezer for approx. 30 minutes.

4: Meanwhile, melt the chocolate in a small bowl in the microwave, stirring every 30 seconds until melted.

5: Fold in the egg whites using a spatula.

6: Remove coconut bites from the freezer and roll each ball in the chocolate until coated. Place balls back onto the tray and place in the fridge to set.

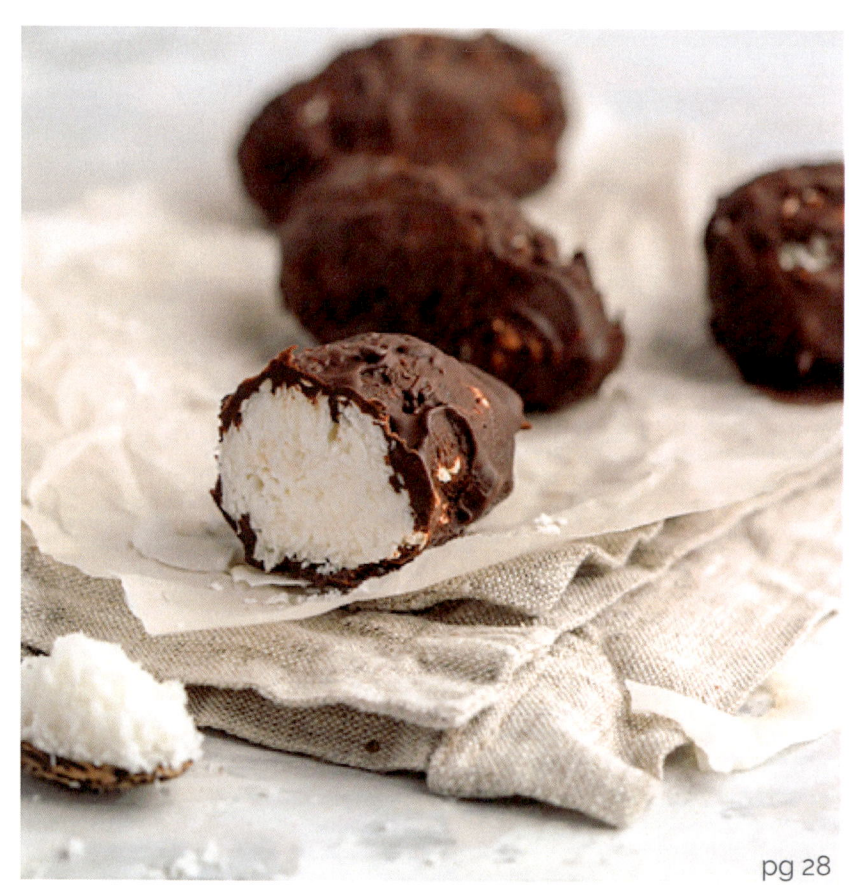

Nutrition Facts

Amount per
1 serving (1.2 oz) — 34 g

Calories 116 — From Fat 72

% Daily Value*

- **Total Fat** 8.5g — 13%
- Saturated Fat 7.4g — 37%
- Trans Fat 0g
- **Cholesterol** 0mg — 0%
- **Sodium** 77mg — 3%
- **Total Carbohydrates** 11g — 4%
- Dietary Fiber 1g — 4%
- Sugars 9g
- **Protein** 1g — 2%

Vitamin A 0% • Vitamin C 0%
Calcium 0% • Iron 3%

* Percent Daily Values are based on 2000 calorie diet. Your Daily Values may be higher or lower depending on your calorie needs.

HappyForks.com

Chocolate Coated Meringues

Yield: Makes approx. 12

Ingredients

4 Egg whites

225g Powdered stevia

1 tsps. Cream of tartar

100g Sugar-free dark chocolate

DIRECTIONS

1: Beat egg whites until stiff.

2: Add powdered stevia a little at a time and the cream of tartar. Beat until powdered stevia is dissolved and the meringue mixture is stiff and glossy. Add sugar to make this step easier.

3: Using a piping bag and a 1cm nozzle pipe rosettes or mounds onto a lined baking tray.

4: Cook in preheated oven 140°C for one hour and then turn off oven and leave for another hour to allow meringues to dry out.

5: Melt 100g sugar free dark chocolate in a heat-proof bowl on high for one minute in a microwave.

6: Using a pastry brush coat meringues with chocolate and set aside to harden chocolate.

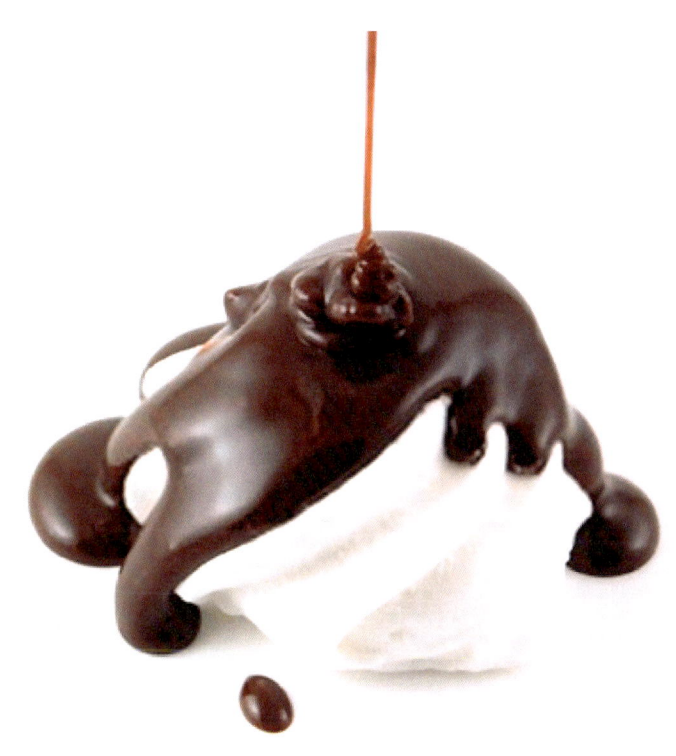

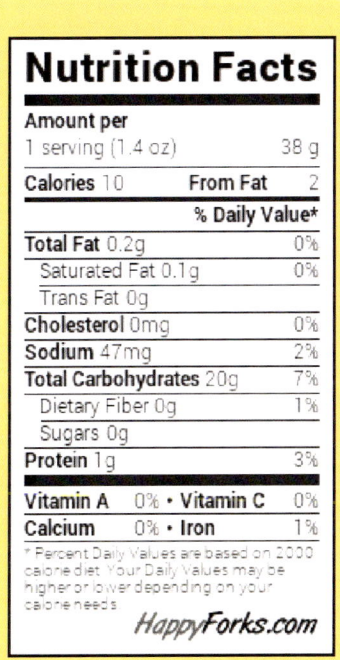

Chocolate & Walnut Slice

Yield: Makes approx. 6 squares

Ingredients

½ cup Chopped dates
½ cup Water
100g Sugar free dark chocolate
1 cup Almond meal
1 tsps. Baking powder
½ cup Powdered stevia
½ tsps. Vanilla essence
½ cup Walnuts (*chopped*)
¼ cup Coconut milk

DIRECTIONS

1: Bring dates and water to the boil in a saucepan, reduce heat. Simmer until pureed.

2: Transfer to a large bowl. Add all other ingredients except chocolate.

3: Break chocolate into pieces and place in a heat proof microwave container. Cook on high for one minute until chocolate is runny.

4: Blend chocolate into the mixture and mix well.

5: Pour into a greased and lined 18 x 28cm slab tin.

6: Bake in a moderate oven at 180°C for 20 minutes or until firm when touched.

7: Allow to cool, then cut into small squares.

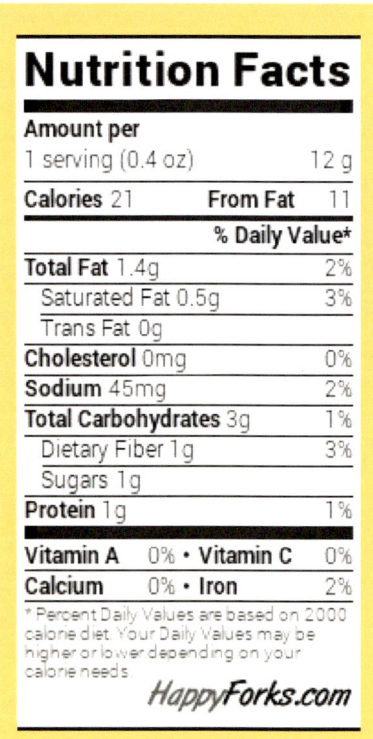

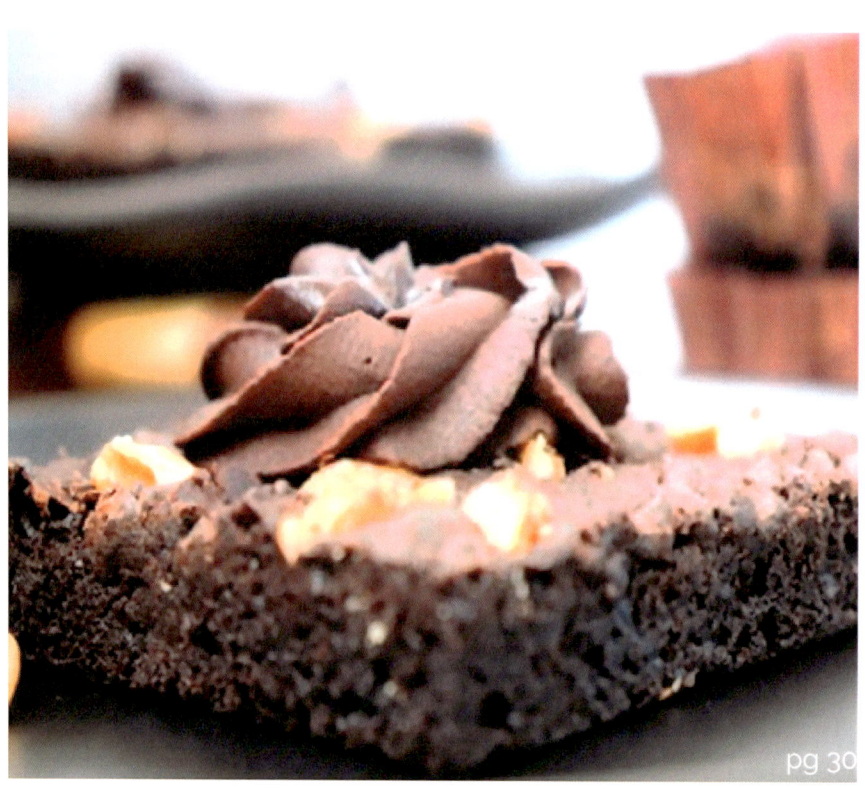

Chocolate Peanut Slice

Yield: Makes Approx. 12

Ingredients

125g Butter
¼ cup Stevia
1 cup Peanut butter
1 Egg
1 cup Almond flour
1 tsps. Baking powder
150g Sugar-free milk chocolate

DIRECTIONS

1: Melt butter, stevia and peanut butter in a saucepan large enough to mix all the ingredients.

2: Add egg and beat with a wooden spoon to combine.

3: Sift almond flour and baking powder into the saucepan.

4: well until combined.

5: Pour into an 18 x 28cm lined, slice tin.

6: Bake at 180°C for 20 minutes.

7: When cold, ice with melted chocolate.

8: To melt chocolate - break into pieces and using a microwave proof jug heat on high for approx. 1 minute.

Nutrition Facts

Amount per
1 serving (2.1 oz)   58 g
Calories 131   From Fat   96
                        % Daily Value*
Total Fat 10.7g   16%
 Saturated Fat 4.6g   23%
 Trans Fat 0g
Cholesterol 63mg   21%
Sodium 524mg   22%
Total Carbohydrates 12g   4%
 Dietary Fiber 1g   3%
 Sugars 4g
Protein 3g   6%

Vitamin A   4% • Vitamin C   0%
Calcium   1% • Iron   5%
* Percent Daily Values are based on 2000 calorie diet. Your Daily Values may be higher or lower depending on your calorie needs.
HappyForks.com

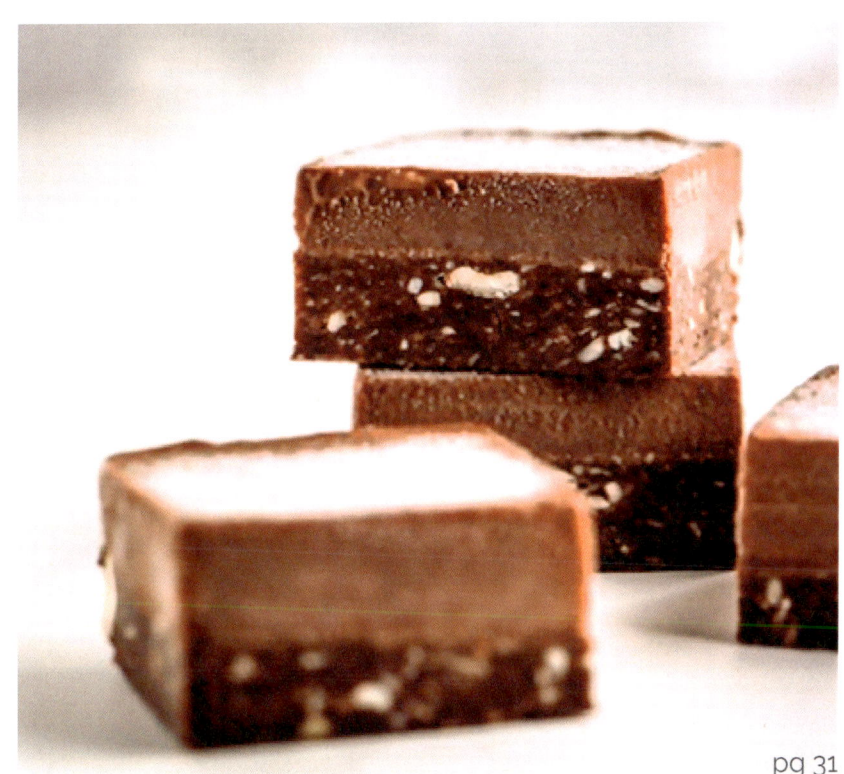

Chocolate Caramel Slice

Yield: Makes Approx. 18 Slices

Ingredients

Base:
- 1 ¼ cup Almond flour
- 5 Tbsp Shredded coconut
- 30g Butter, melted
- 50g Almond butter
- 1-5 drops Liquid stevia

Caramel layer
- 50g Butter
- 70g Thick cream or coconut cream
- 2 heaped tbsp Almond butter
- 2 tbsp Sukrin syrup
- Pinch of Salt

Chocolate layer
- 100g Sugar Free dark chocolate

DIRECTIONS

1: To make base layer, add all ingredients to a food processor and pulse until combined. The mixture should appear crumbly but should hold when pressed together between the fingers.

2: Press firmly into a loaf pan or small slice pan (15 x 23 cms). Place in the freezer while you make the caramel layer.

3: To make the caramel, melt the butter in a small saucepan over medium to low heat, stirring constantly, until it starts to brown.

4: Add the remaining ingredients and stir until combined, then reduce heat until just simmering, and cook 5-10 minutes or until it starts to thicken. Note that it will continue to thicken as it cools. Pour over the base layer and spread evenly. Return to the freezer while you make the chocolate layer.

5: Melt the chocolate in the microwave for approx. 1 min, and when runny, pour onto the solidified caramel layer. Spread evenly. Place back in the freezer for at least an hour to set.

6: Once set, cut into squares or bars, and store in an airtight container in the fridge.

Nutrition Facts

Amount per
1 serving (0.7 oz) — 21 g

Calories 62	From Fat	42
		% Daily Value*
Total Fat 4.9g		8%
Saturated Fat 2.7g		14%
Trans Fat 0g		
Cholesterol 0mg		0%
Sodium 46mg		2%
Total Carbohydrates 6g		2%
Dietary Fiber 1g		5%
Sugars 3g		
Protein 1g		2%
Vitamin A 0% • Vitamin C		0%
Calcium 1% • Iron		4%

* Percent Daily Values are based on 2000 calorie diet. Your Daily Values may be higher or lower depending on your calorie needs.

HappyForks.com

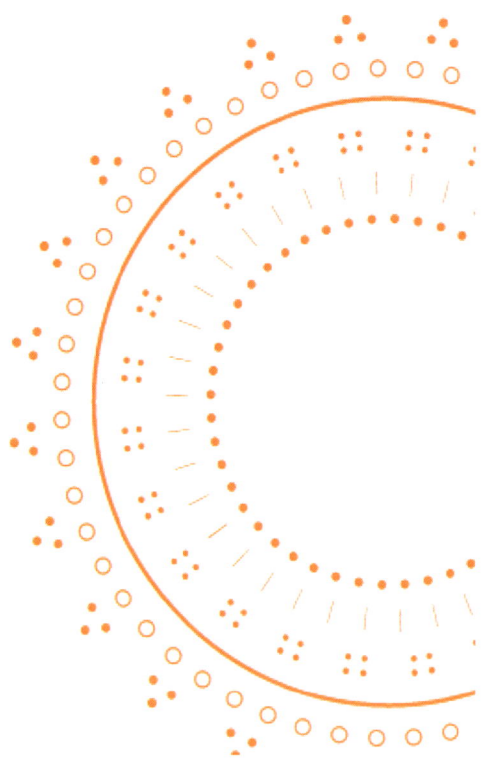

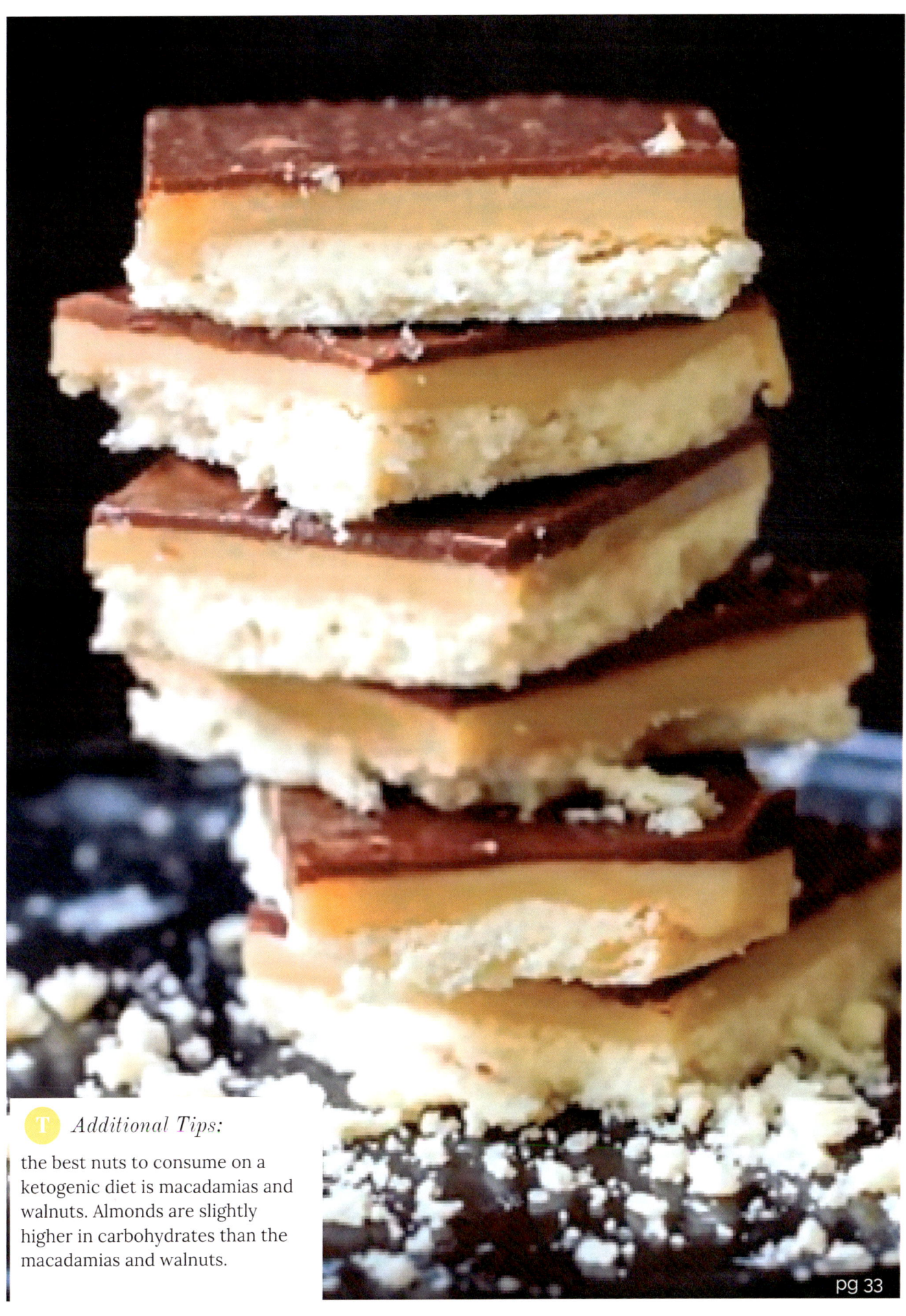

> **T** *Additional Tips:*
> the best nuts to consume on a ketogenic diet is macadamias and walnuts. Almonds are slightly higher in carbohydrates than the macadamias and walnuts.

Chocolate Nutty Bars

Yield: Makes Approx. 12 bars

Ingredients

⅓ cup Sukrin Gold Fibre Syrup
2 Tbsp Coconut oil
(*Extra virgin organic*)
Pinch Pink Himalayan salt
1 cup Almonds,
(*coarsely chopped*)
1 cup Pecans or walnuts,
(*coarsely chopped*)
1 cup Pumpkin seeds,
(*coarsely chopped*)
1 Tbsp Chia seeds
2 Tbsp Desiccated coconut
1 tsps. Ground cinnamon
200g Dark chocolate
(*Sugar free*)

DIRECTIONS

1: Grease and line an 8-inch square baking tin with baking paper and set aside.

2: Sukrin Gold Fibre Syrup , coconut oil and a pinch of salt in a small saucepan over medium heat for about 10 minutes until it begins to thicken and turn a rich, golden caramel colour (keep an eye on the heat so that it doesn't bubble over suddenly).

3: Fold in the chopped nuts, cinnamon seeds and coconut and stir until evenly coated.

4: Remove from heat and pour into the lined baking pan. Cover with another sheet of baking paper and press down firmly – using a tea towel if needed to protect your fingers from the heat to form an even layer. Refrigerate until hardened.

5: Cut into squares with a sharp knife and keep refrigerated until you're ready to dip in the melted chocolate.

6: Melt chocolate in the microwave in a heat proof container for approx. 1 min until runny. stir with a metal spoon until smooth.

7: Dip one end or corner of each square into melted chocolate and sprinkle with a few flakes of salt before placing on a baking paper lined tray to set in the fridge.

8: After an hour, the bars will be ready to enjoy.

Nutrition Facts

Amount per 48 g
1 serving (1.7 oz)
Calories 161
From fat 102
HappyForks.com

Amount	% Daily Value*	Amount	% Daily Value*
Total Fat 12.1g	19%	Total Carbohydrates 13g	4%
Saturated 1.8g	9%	Dietary Fiber 2g	8%
Trans Fat 0g		Sugars 8g	
Cholesterol 0mg	0%	Protein 5g	9%
Sodium 98mg	4%		
Calcium 2% • Iron 8%		Vitamin A 0% • Vitamin C 1%	

* Percent Daily Values are based on 2000 calorie diet. Your Daily Values may be higher or lower depending on your calorie needs.

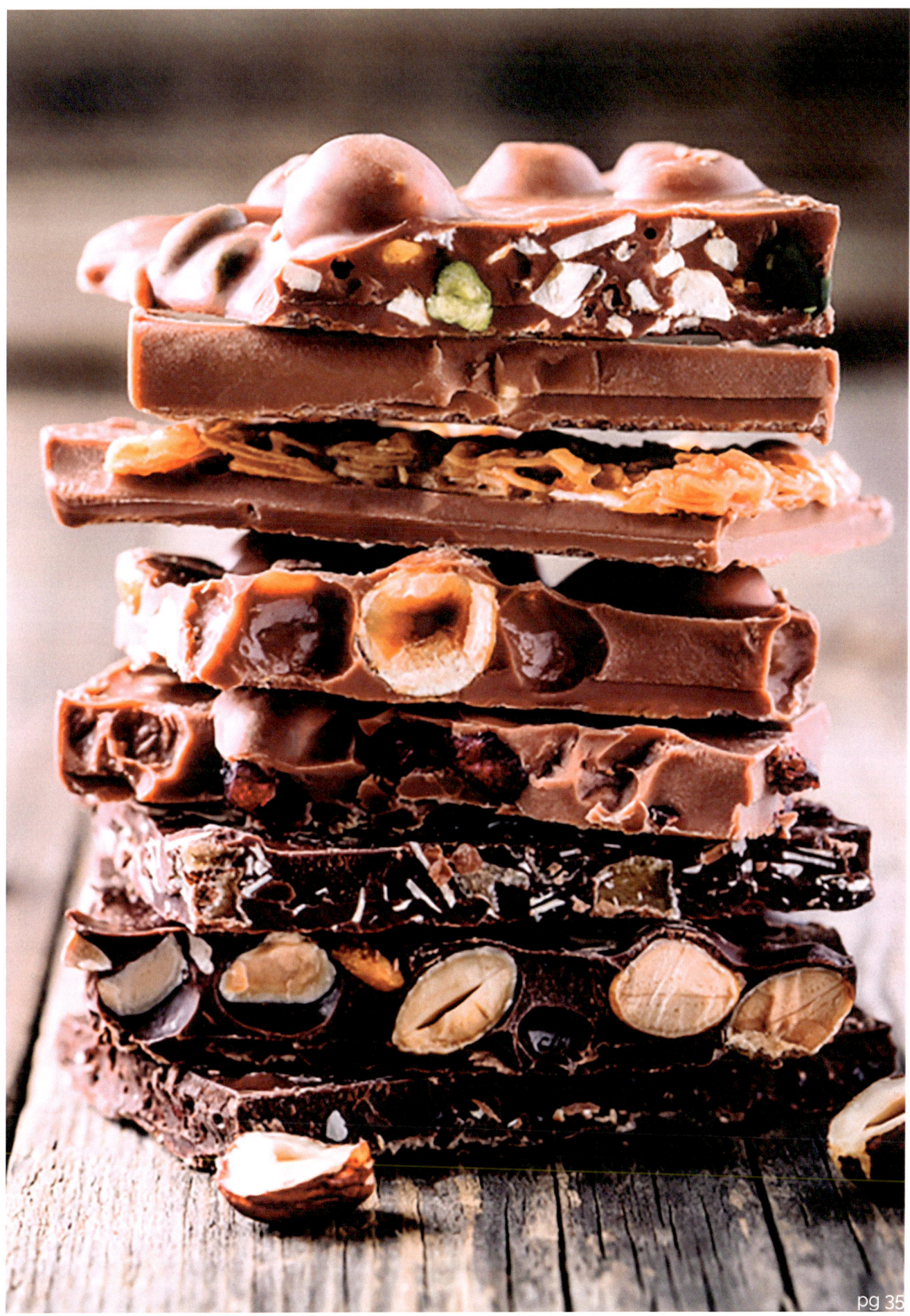

pg 35

Double Chocolate Brownies

Yield: Makes 12 brownies

Ingredients

150g Butter softened (*organic/grass fed e.g. Kerry Gold*)
¾ cup Powdered Stevia
½ cup Coconut cream
4 Free range eggs, (*lightly whisked*)
1 cup Almond meal
1 cup Cocoa powder
Pinch Pink Himalayan salt
½ cup Coconut flour
1 Tbsp Melted Coconut oil
300g Sugar-free dark chocolate
½ cup Walnuts/ Pistachios

DIRECTIONS

1: Pre-heat oven to 180c and line a 20cm x 15cm baking dish with baking paper.

2: Mix the butter and stevia together with a wooden spoon until light and creamy. Add the coconut cream and eggs and mix well.

3: Combine the almond meal, cacao powder and coconut flour together in a small bowl with a pinch of pink Himalayan salt, before adding to the wet ingredients and stirring with a wooden spoon until a smooth batter is formed.

4: Fold through the sugar free dark chocolate chunks and walnuts or pistachios.

5: Pour the batter into the prepared baking dish and bake for 45 minutes, or until the centre is slightly firm.

6: Allow to cool before cutting into squares and serving

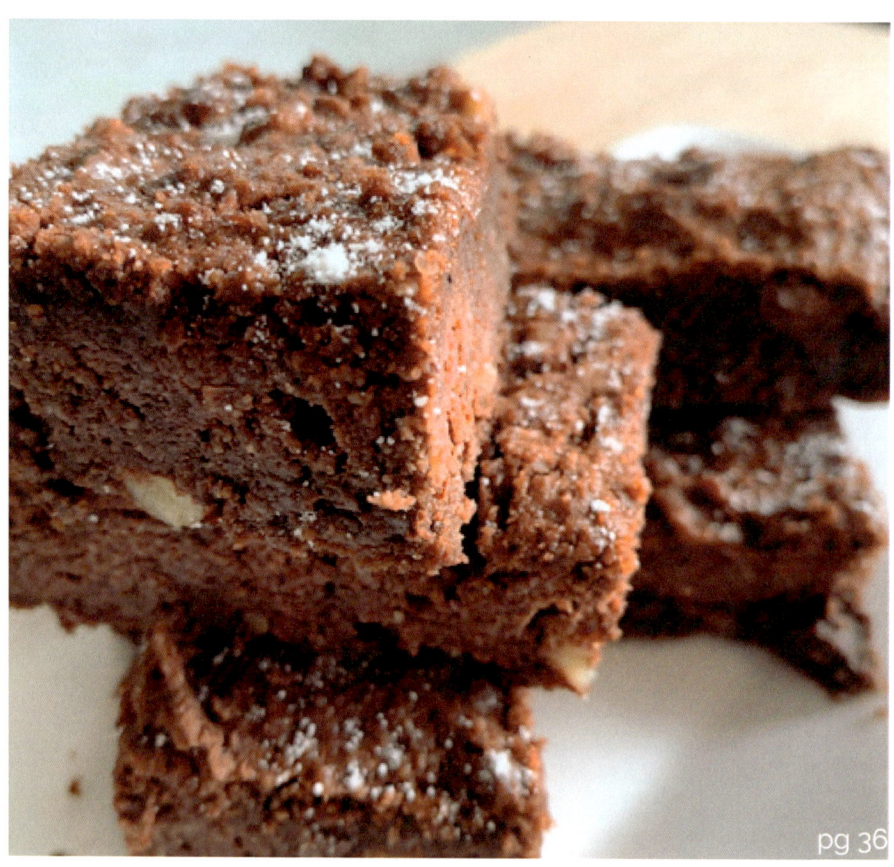

My 'Turkish Delight'

Yield: Makes 36

Ingredients

400ml Water
5 Medium fresh strawberries, (*hulled & very finely diced*)
8 tsps. Liquid stevia
1 tsps. Cream of tartar
1 Tbsp Rosewater
¼ tsps. Vanilla extract
1 tsps. Beetroot powder
12 Gelatine leaves

Chocolate coating:
100g Sugar-free milk chocolate, (*chopped into small pieces*)
3 tsps. Butter

DIRECTIONS

1: Place the gelatine leaves in a small bowl of water to soften.

2: Place water, finely chopped strawberries, granulated sweetener & cream of tartar in a medium pot and bring to a gentle simmer, stirring until the strawberries have infused into the water and the sweetener has dissolved.

3: Remove pot from the heat and stir in rosewater, vanilla & beetroot powder. Pour mixture through a fine sieve into a medium bowl.

4: Squeeze out the excess water from the gelatine and place the softened leaves into the mix and whisk vigorously to combine.

5: Pour mixture into prepared tin and place in the fridge to set – about 1 hour. Once set, remove and cut into bars (just like a Turkish Delight chocolate bar).

6: Melt chocolate & butter in a small bowl set over a pot of simmering water, stirring together until smooth. Allow chocolate to cool a little, then dip Turkish Delight bars in the melted chocolate before transferring to a baking paper lined plate to set in the fridge.

7: Keep stored in an airtight container in the fridge for up to a week

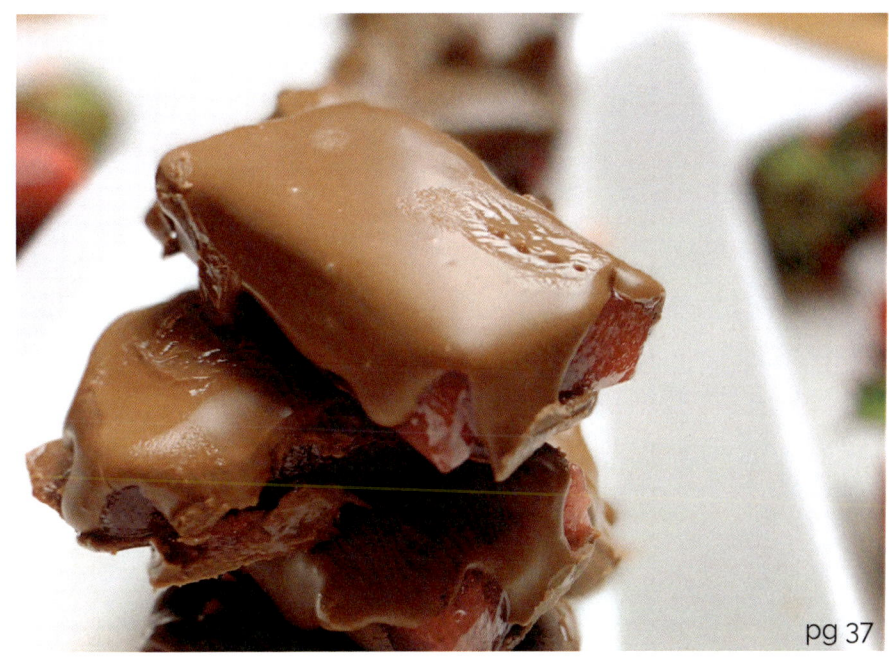

Nutrition Facts

Amount per 1 serving (0.7 oz) — 19 g

Calories 6	From Fat 3	
		% Daily Value*
Total Fat 0.3g		1%
Saturated Fat 0.2g		1%
Trans Fat 0g		
Cholesterol 0mg		0%
Sodium 13mg		1%
Total Carbohydrates 1g		0%
Dietary Fiber 0g		0%
Sugars 0g		
Protein 0g		0%
Vitamin A 0%	Vitamin C	2%
Calcium 0%	Iron	1%

* Percent Daily Values are based on 2000 calorie diet. Your Daily Values may be higher or lower depending on your calorie needs

Chocolate Swirl Muffins

Yield: 10 muffins

Ingredients

- 125g Butter
- ½ cup Powdered stevia
- 2 Eggs
- 1 ¾ cups Almond Flour
- 2 tsps. Baking powder
- ⅔ cup Coconut milk
- ½ cup Sugar-free dark chocolate (*melted*)

DIRECTIONS

1: Preheat oven 180°C and line 10-hole muffin tin with patty cases.

2: Cream the softened butter and sugar until light and fluffy.

3: Add eggs one at a time and mix well.

4: Sift the almond flour and baking powder.

5: Pour in coconut milk and mix all ingredients together.

6: Melt chocolate in a microwave and swirl though mixture.

7: Using a spoon take mixture and place into patty cases.

8: Cook in oven for 15-20 minutes until muffins are cooked.

9: Cool on wire rack.

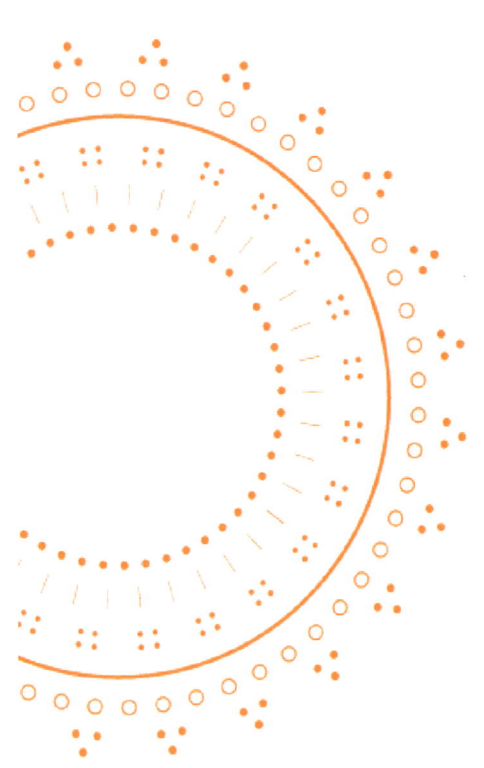

Nutrition Facts

Amount per 1 serving (2.2 oz) 62 g

Calories 146
From fat 122

HappyForks.com

	Amount	% Daily Value*	Amount	% Daily Value*
Total Fat	13.9g	21%	Total Carbohydrates 6g	2%
Saturated	8.8g	44%	Dietary Fiber 2g	9%
Trans Fat	0g		Sugars 1g	
Cholesterol	137mg	46%	Protein 4g	8%
Sodium	128mg	5%		
Calcium	2% • Iron 11%		Vitamin A 6% • Vitamin C	1%

* Percent Daily Values are based on 2000 calorie diet. Your Daily Values may be higher or lower depending on your calorie needs.

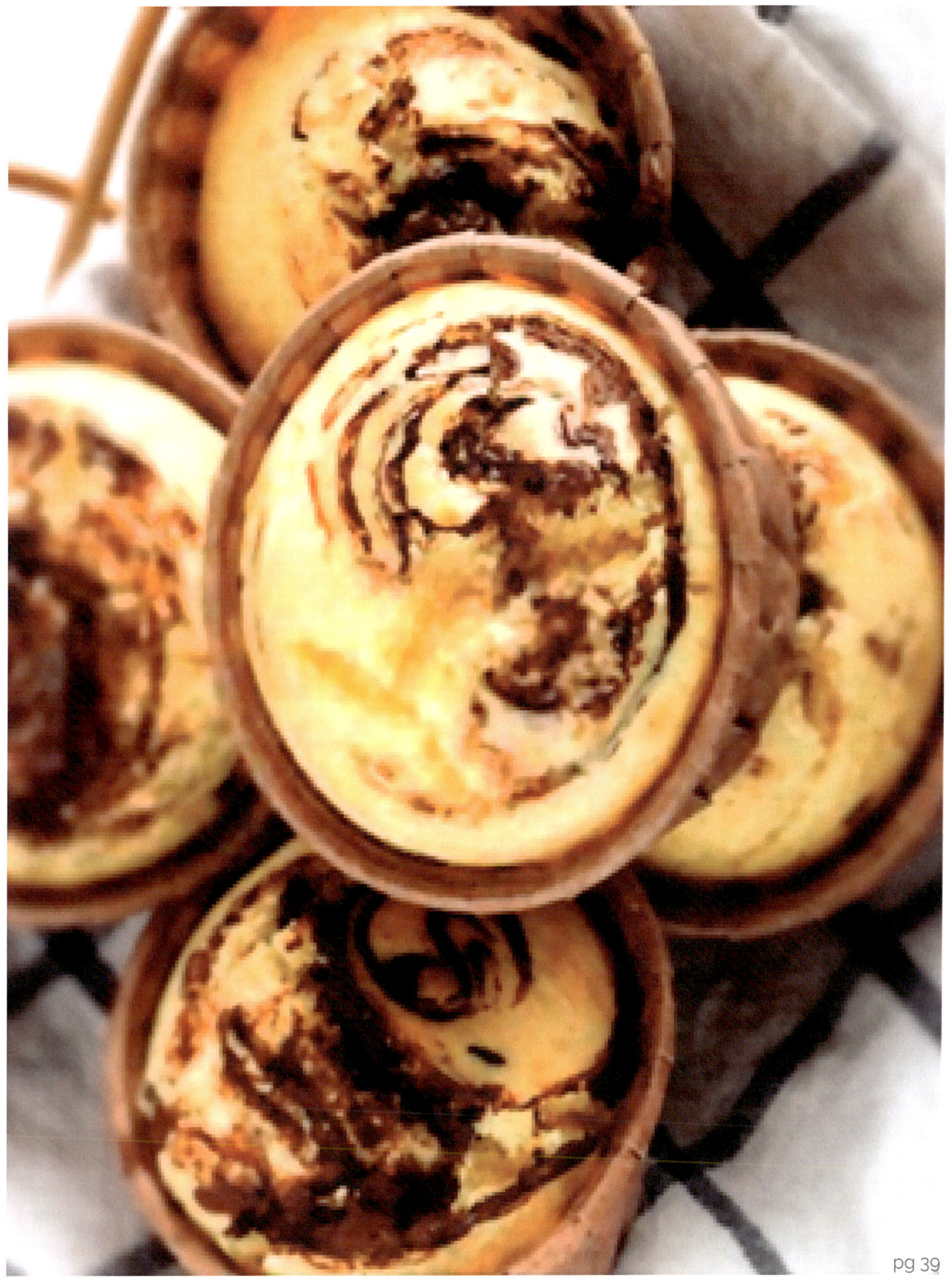

Chocolate- Zucchini Muffins

Yield: Makes 24 muffins

Ingredients

- 2 cups Shredded zucchini
- 3 Eggs
- ¼ cup Powdered stevia
- ¾ cup Plain Greek yogurt
- 2 tsps. Vanilla extract
- 2 cups Almond meal
- ⅔ cup Unsweetened cocoa powder
- ½ tsps. Baking powder
- 1 tsps. Salt
- ½ cup Sugar-free dark chocolate

DIRECTIONS

1: Preheat oven to 170°C

2: In a large bowl, mix shredded zucchini, eggs, stevia, yogurt and vanilla; set aside.

3: In a separate bowl, mix almond meal, cocoa powder, baking powder and salt.

4: Add dry ingredients to the wet ingredients and mix until just combined.

5: Melt the chocolate in a heat proof container in the microwave for approximately 1 min. Gently fold the chocolate into the rest of the mixture.

6: Spoon mixture into 24 prepared muffin cups, about 3/4 full, and bake for about 25 minutes or until a skewer inserted comes out clean.

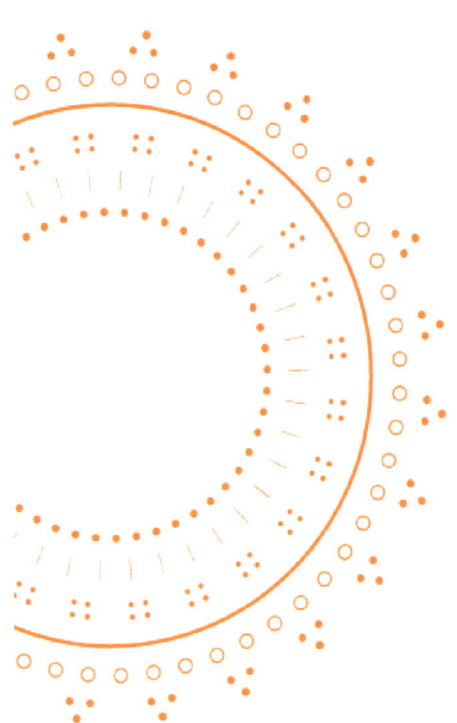

Nutrition Facts

Amount per 1 serving (1.4 oz) 39 g

Calories 50
From fat 25

HappyForks.com

Amount	% Daily Value*	Amount	% Daily Value*
Total Fat 2.9g	5%	Total Carbohydrates 8g	3%
Saturated 1.3g	6%	Dietary Fiber 4g	14%
Trans Fat 0g		Sugars 1g	
Cholesterol 78mg	26%	Protein 4g	8%
Sodium 154mg	6%		
Calcium 3% • Iron 13%		Vitamin A 1% • Vitamin C 1%	

* Percent Daily Values are based on 2000 calorie diet. Your Daily Values may be higher or lower depending on your calorie needs.

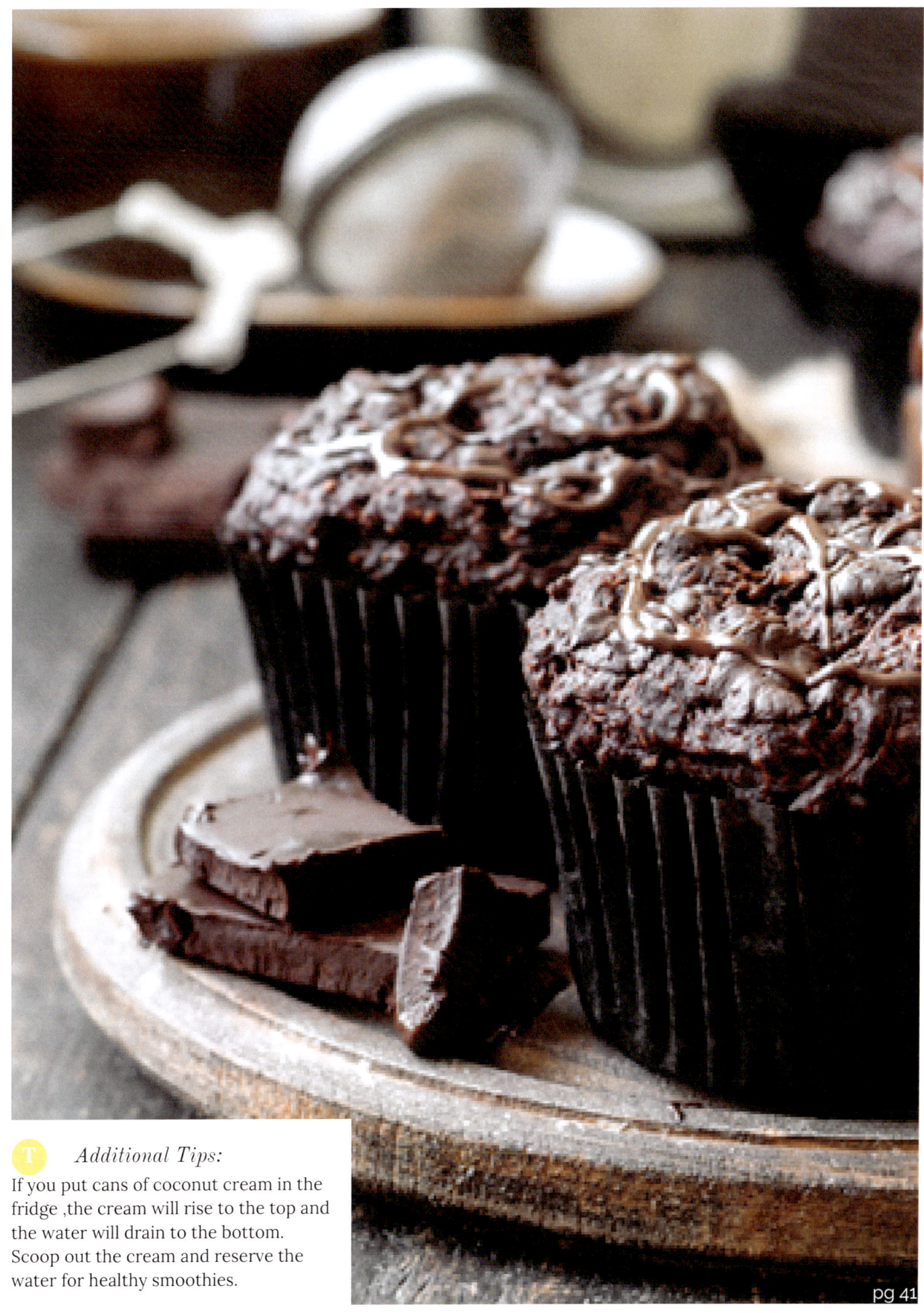

T *Additional Tips:*
If you put cans of coconut cream in the fridge, the cream will rise to the top and the water will drain to the bottom. Scoop out the cream and reserve the water for healthy smoothies.

White Chocolate Friands

Yield: Serves - 12

Ingredients

1 cup Almond flour/
(*or almond meal*)
1 ½ cup Icing sugar (sukrin)
or substitute finely powdered stevia
½ cup Coconut flour
2 Tbsp Cocoa
100g Sugar-free white chocolate
(*finely grated*)
5 Egg whites
180g Butter

DIRECTIONS

1: Sift combined sugar-free icing sugar, almond flour, coconut flour and cocoa into a large bowl.

2: Add the grated white chocolate and mix well.

3: In a separate bowl, beat egg whites until soft peaks form.

4: Melt butter in the microwave for about 1 minute.

5: Add to dry ingredients and mix to combine.

6: Gently fold in egg whites.

7: Spoon mixture into lightly greased or sprayed friand moulds until ¼ full.

8: Bake in a hot oven 200°C for 15-20 minutes or until firm and cooked when tested with a skewer.

9: Cool for 5 minutes in pan before transferring to a wire rack to cool completely.

10: To serve dust with sugar free icing sugar or serve with strawberries and cream.

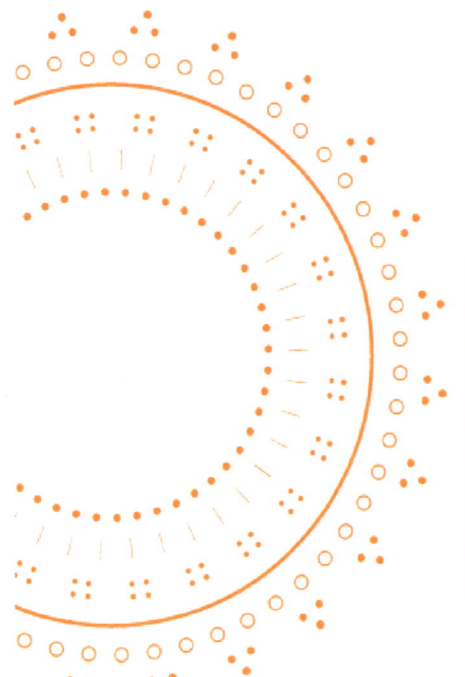

Nutrition Facts

Amount per 74 g
1 serving (2.6 oz)

Calories 119
From fat 87

HappyForks.com

	Amount	% Daily Value*	Amount	% Daily Value*
Total Fat 9.7g		15%	**Total Carbohydrates** 5g	2%
Saturated 6.3g		31%	Dietary Fiber 1g	3%
Trans Fat 0g			Sugars 3g	
Cholesterol 17mg		6%	**Protein** 4g	8%
Sodium 154mg		6%		
Calcium 6% • **Iron** 3%			**Vitamin A** 6% • **Vitamin C** 0%	

* Percent Daily Values are based on 2000 calorie diet. Your Daily Values may be higher or lower depending on your calorie needs

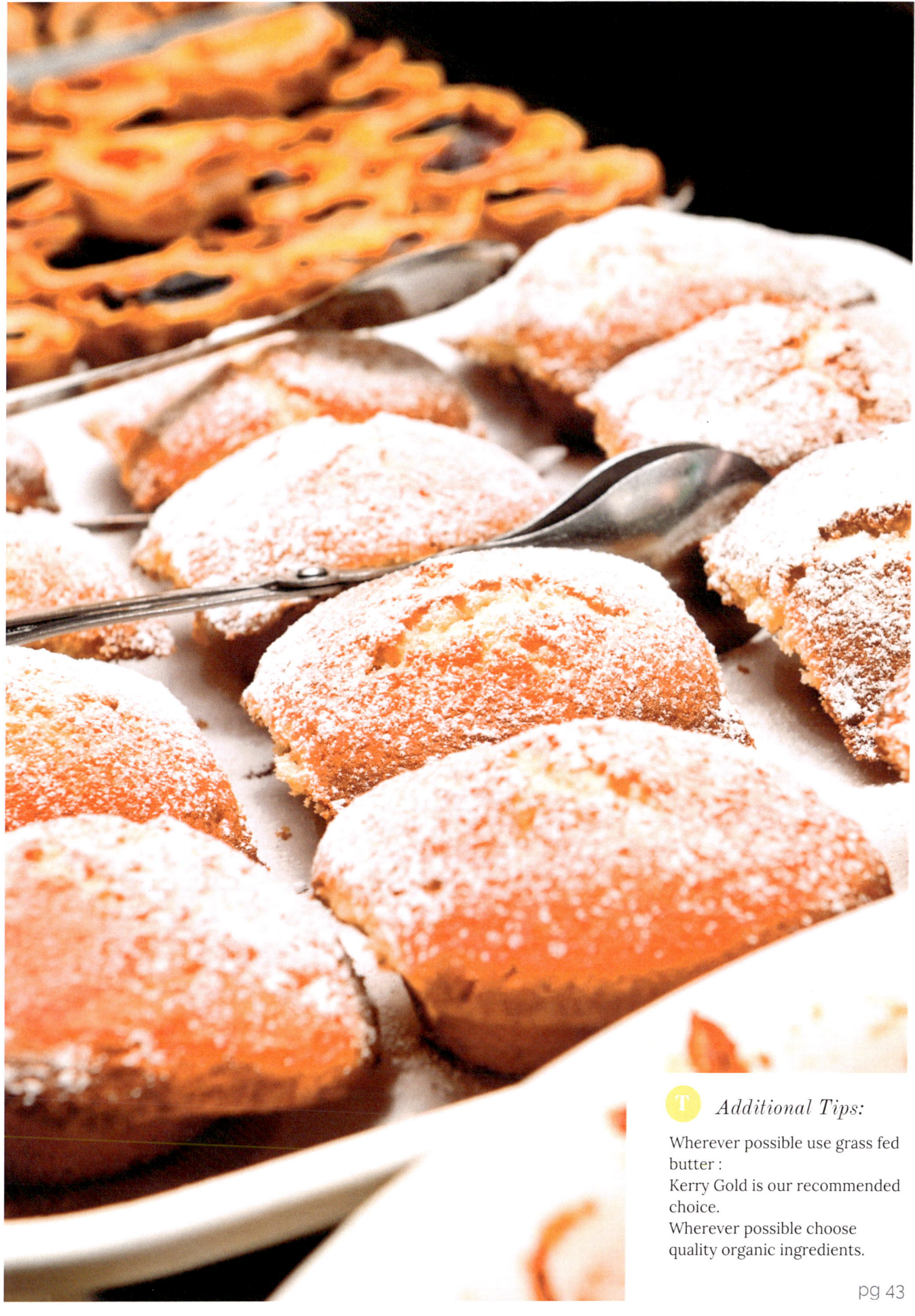

Additional Tips:

Wherever possible use grass fed butter :
Kerry Gold is our recommended choice.
Wherever possible choose quality organic ingredients.

Mmmmm......Donuts

Yield: Serves 12 medium sized donuts

Ingredients

250g Cream Cheese
(*room temperature*)

6 large Eggs

2 tsps. Vanilla Extract

8 Tbsp Almond Flour

4 Tbsp Coconut Flour

8 Tbsp Stevia
(*Finely Ground*)

1 tsps. Cinnamon powder

Glaze

200g Sugar-free dark chocolate

1 tsps. Coconut oil

DIRECTIONS

1: Add the eggs, cream cheese, stevia and vanilla extract into a mixing bowl. Blend with an electric mixer until smooth.

2: Add the sifted almond flour, coconut flour, cinnamon powder and baking powder. Blend until well combined.

3: Let the batter sit in the fridge for at least 30 mins or overnight to allow the batter to rest and thicken.

4: To cook your donuts – All you need is a donut ring shaped non-stick baking tray. Pre-heat your oven to approx. 180 degree C.

5: Fill the donut batter into the donut tray and place in the middle of the oven for approximately 12-15mins (*depending on your oven.*) They will start to rise, and you should have that beautiful familiar cinnamon donut smell.

6: Melt your sugar free dark chocolate in the microwave for approx 1 min. Add the coconut oil and mix until smooth.

7: Remove your donuts from the oven and allow to cool on a wire rack.

8: Pour the melted chocaolate icing over the donuts and allow to set.

9: Donuts will last approx 2 weeks in a covered container in the fridge.

Nutrition Facts

Amount per
1 serving (2.4 oz) — 69 g

Calories 129 — From Fat 89

	% Daily Value*
Total Fat 10.2g	16%
Saturated Fat 2.3g	12%
Trans Fat 0g	
Cholesterol 312mg	104%
Sodium 93mg	4%
Total Carbohydrates 14g	5%
Dietary Fiber 1g	5%
Sugars 1g	
Protein 7g	13%
Vitamin A 5% • Vitamin C 0%	
Calcium 5% • Iron 10%	

* Percent Daily Values are based on 2000 calorie diet. Your Daily Values may be higher or lower depending on your calorie needs.

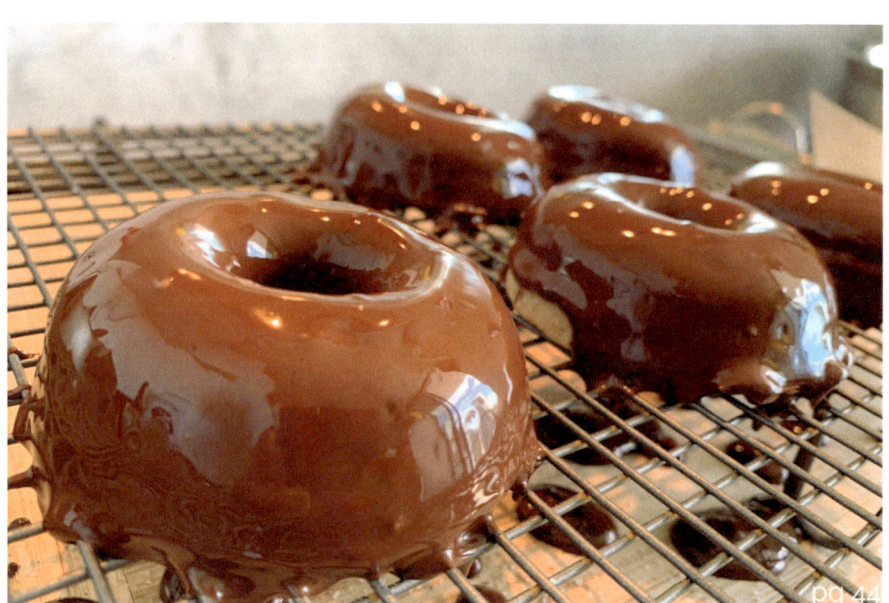

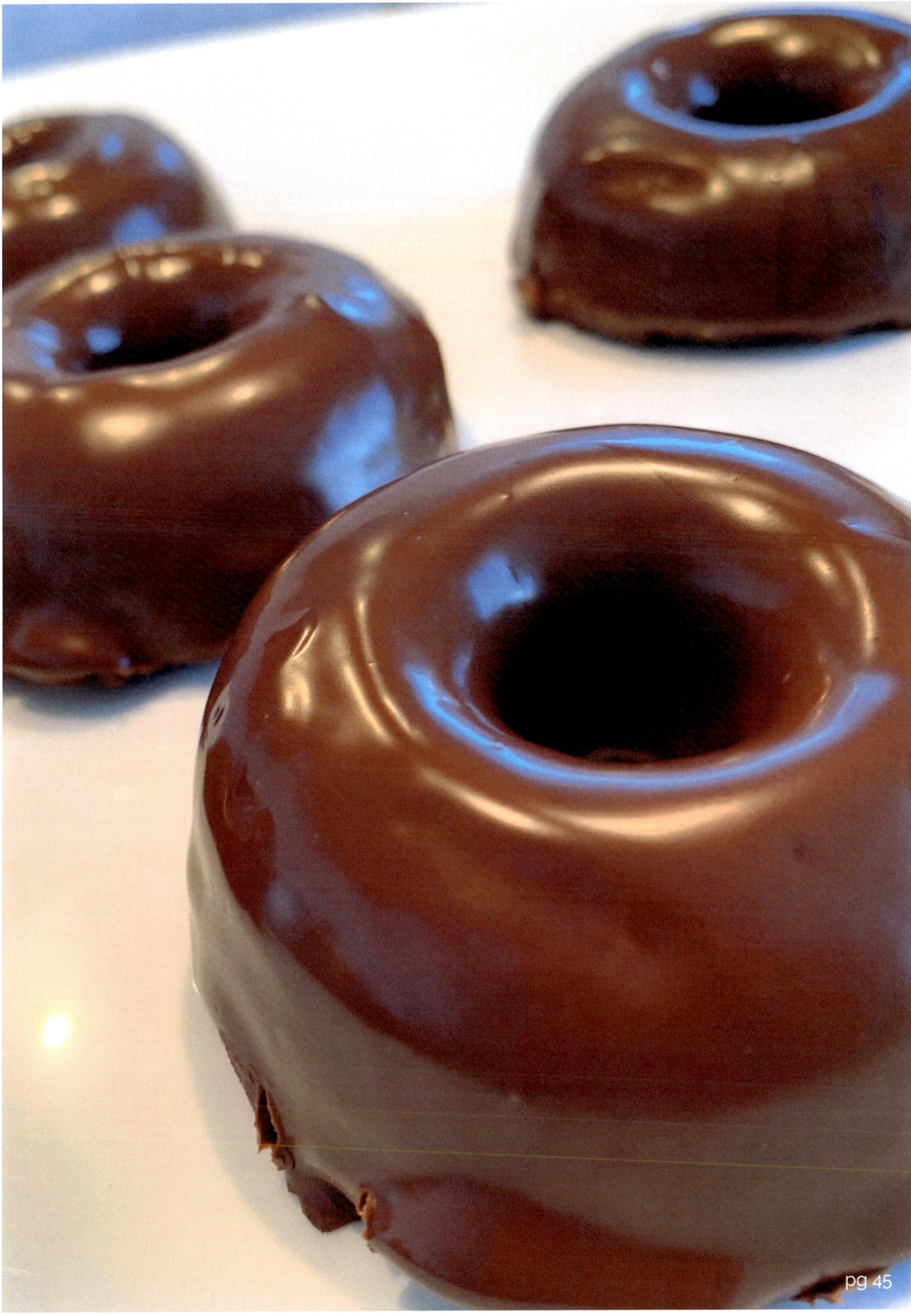

Chocolate Waffles

Yield: Makes 4 waffles

Ingredients

120 g   Cream Cheese
(*room temperature*)
1 Tbsp Butter
1 Tbsp Organic Cocoa powder
1 ½ tsps. Vanilla Extract
1 Tbsp Stevia
4 Tbsp Coconut Flour
1 ½ tsps. Baking Powder

DIRECTIONS

1: Simply add all the ingredients into a food processor or blender and mix to a batter consistency.

2: Let it rest in the fridge whilst you heat up the waffle iron.

3: Ensure you spray your waffle iron with a little oil and then add your waffle batter.

4: Cook as per your waffle iron time or until light and golden.

5: Top with any keto friendly ingredient like whipped cream, Greek yoghurt, sugar free maple syrup or berries.

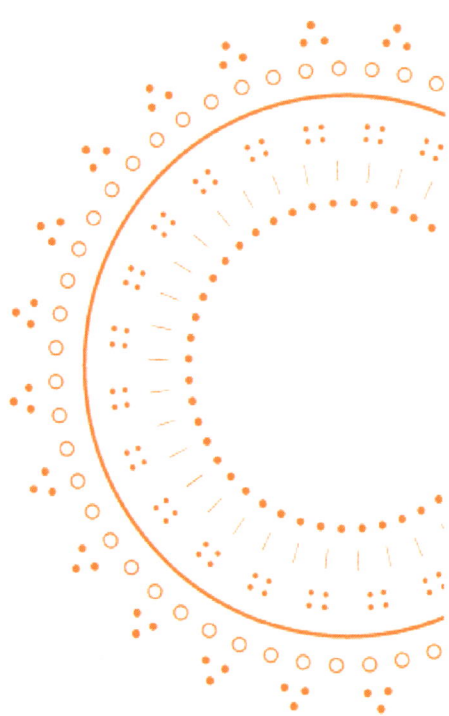

Nutrition Facts

Amount per
1 serving (2.1 oz) — 58 g

Calories 118	From Fat 96
	% Daily Value*
Total Fat 10.7g	16%
Saturated Fat 6.7g	34%
Trans Fat 0g	
Cholesterol 31mg	10%
Sodium 164mg	7%
Total Carbohydrates 8g	3%
Dietary Fiber 1g	2%
Sugars 2g	
Protein 3g	5%
Vitamin A 7% • Vitamin C	1%
Calcium 11% • Iron	4%

* Percent Daily Values are based on 2000 calorie diet. Your Daily Values may be higher or lower depending on your calorie needs.

HappyForks.com

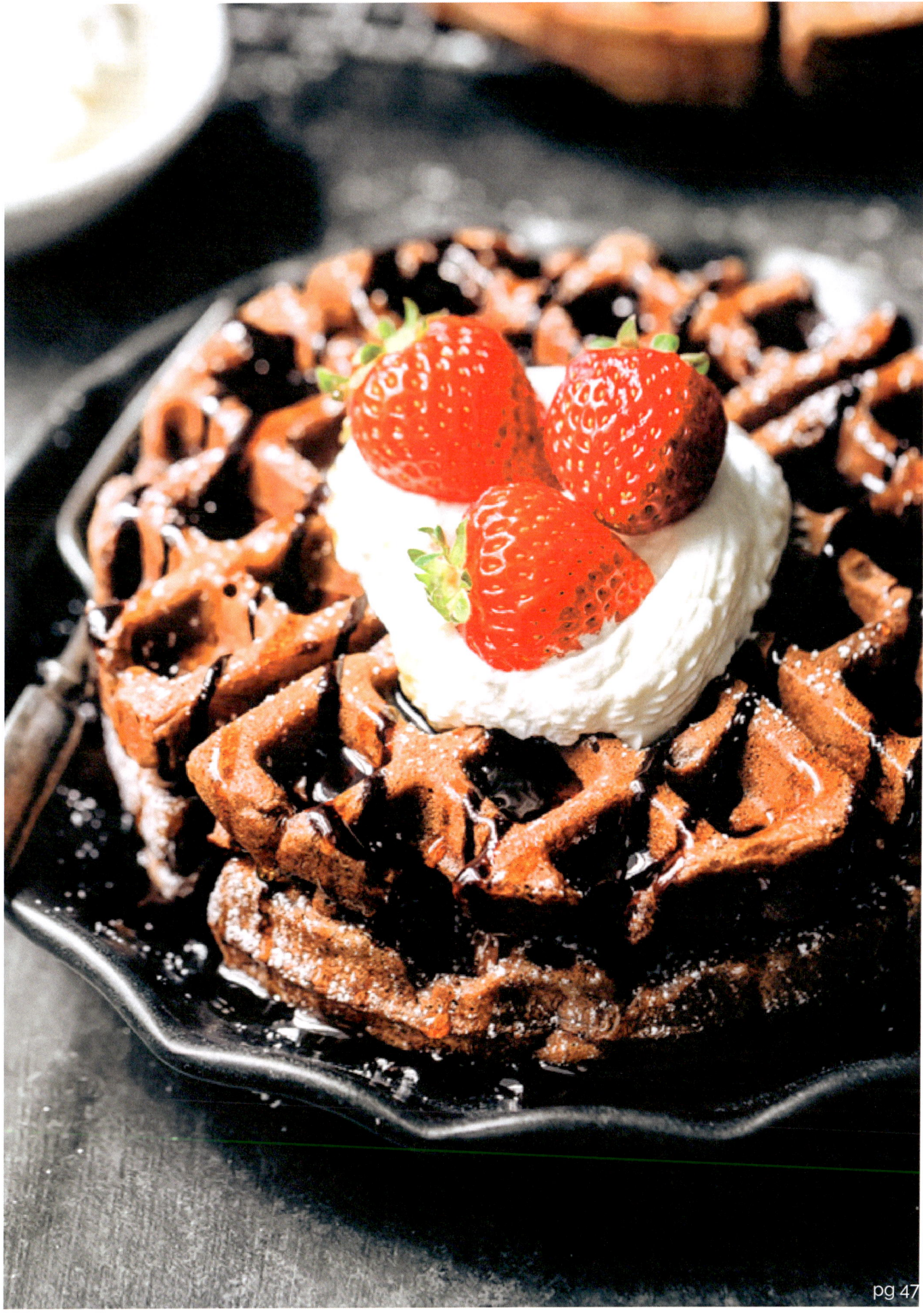

Chocolate Chip Cookies

Yield: Makes Approx. 24 cookies

Ingredients

2 cups Almond meal
⅓ cup Powdered stevia
1 pinch Pink Himalayan salt
1 tsps. Vanilla extract
½ cup Unsalted butter, softened (*use Kerry gold – Grass fed/organic*)
1 Egg free range organic
125g Sugar-free dark chocolate

(*finely chopped into chunks*)

DIRECTIONS

1: Add all the dry ingredients – almond meal – stevia- salt.

2: Add the softened butter – use the '*rubbing method*' to make even crumb like texture.

3: Add vanilla extract and egg and beat until combined.

4: Add the chopped sugar free chocolate to the mixture and combine. Mixture should resemble a dough like texture.

5: Place mixture into baking paper. Roll the baking paper around the dough until you get a sausage like shape. Place in the fridge for about 20-30mins until the dough firms up.

6: Remove from the fridge and slice into biscuits. The cookies will not spread so the size you cut is the size they will be. So cut as thin or as thick as you desire.

7: Cook in a preheated oven at 160°C approx. 15 -20 mins – (varies on your oven) or until golden brown.

8: Cool on wire rack. Enjoy!!

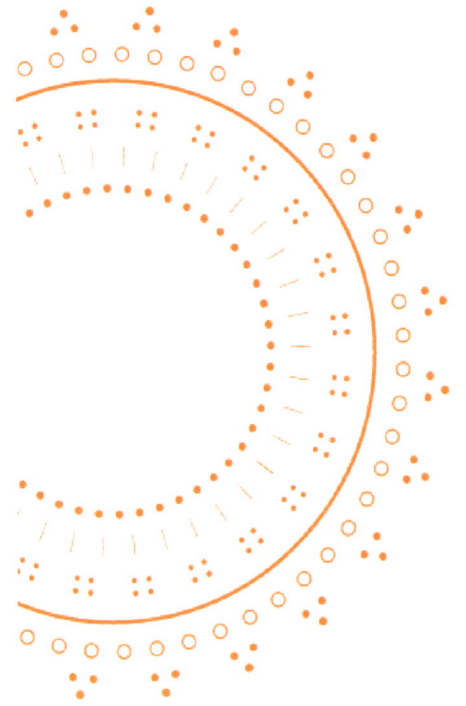

Nutrition Facts

Amount per 25 g
1 serving (0.9 oz)

Calories 86
From fat 45

HappyForks.com

	Amount	% Daily Value*	Amount	% Daily Value*
Total Fat	5.1g	8%	Total Carbohydrates 10g	3%
Saturated	2.9g	15%	Dietary Fiber 1g	6%
Trans Fat	0.2g		Sugars 2g	
Cholesterol	37mg	12%	Protein 2g	3%
Sodium	62mg	3%		
Calcium	1% • Iron	3%	Vitamin A 18% • Vitamin C	8%

* Percent Daily Values are based on 2000 calorie diet. Your Daily Values may be higher or lower depending on your calorie needs.

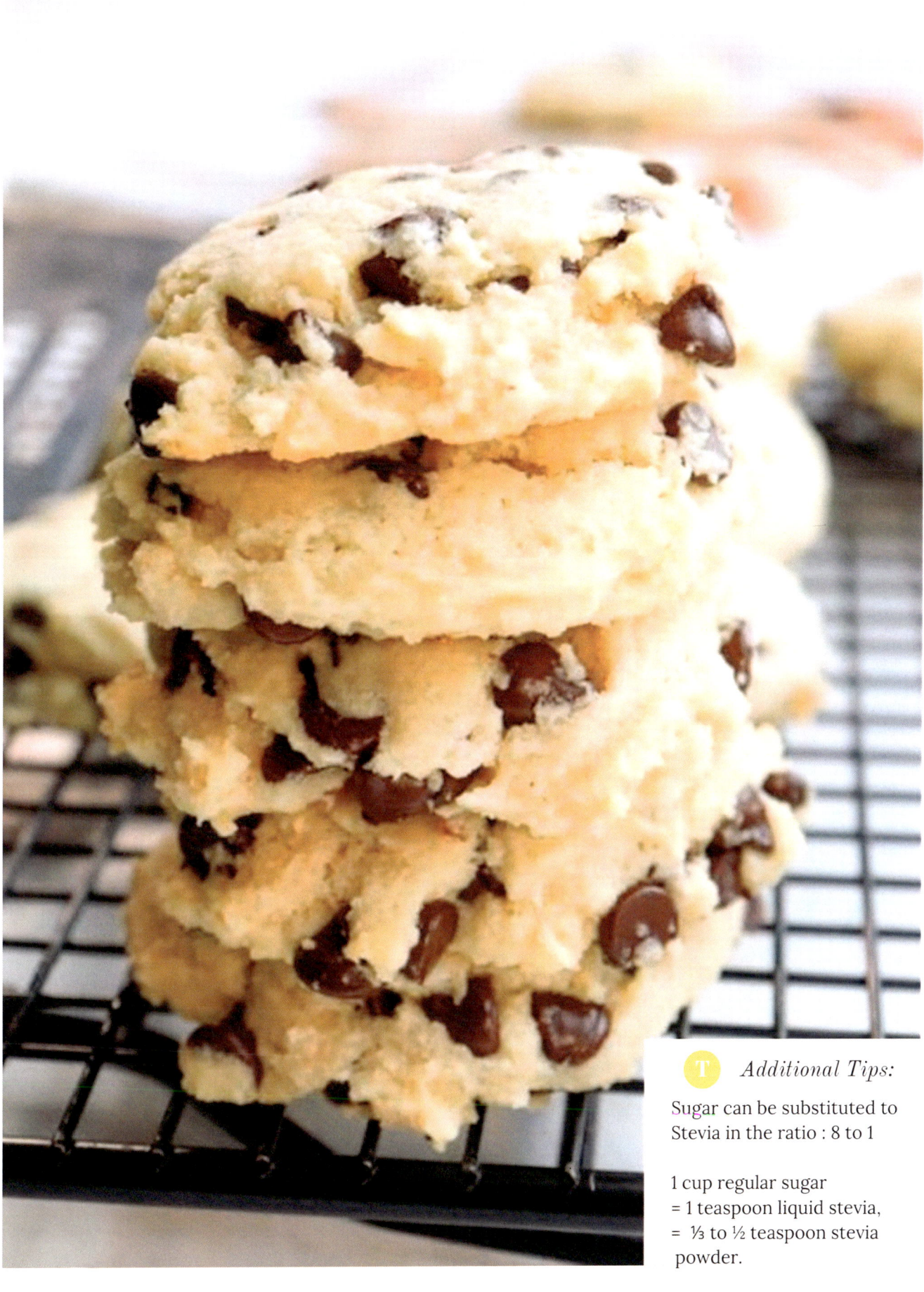

T *Additional Tips:*

Sugar can be substituted to Stevia in the ratio : 8 to 1

1 cup regular sugar
= 1 teaspoon liquid stevia,
= ⅓ to ½ teaspoon stevia powder.

'Choc-Mint Slices'

Yield: makes approx. 12 biscuits

Ingredients

Biscuit

2 cups Almond meal
¼ cup Cocoa powder
1 pinch of Pink Himalayan salt
½ cup Powdered stevia
150g Butter (use Kerry gold – Grass fed/organic)
1 Egg- free range organic

Filling

¼ cup Thick Cream
2 tablespoons melted coconut oil
2 tablespoons Liquid Stevia
¼ tsps. Xantham gum
½ tsps. Peppermint essence (to taste)

Topping

200g Sugar-free dark chocolate
40g Butter

DIRECTIONS

Make the peppermint filing :

1: Mix the cream, liquid stevia and peppermint drops and xanthan gum whisk until thick. Heat the coconut oil until melted but not hot.

2: Pour in the coconut oil into the cream mixture and whisk well. Set aside in the refrigerator.

Make the biscuits

1: Add the almond meal, cocoa, stevia, salt, all together.

2: Add the softened butter and use the rubbing method to blend the mix until it resembles breadcrumbs.

3: Then add the egg mix until it combines and comes away from the bowl and resembles a thick dough.

4: Place on baking paper or glad wrap and roll into a sausage like shape. Place this is in the fridge for half an hour or so to set.

5: Remove the fridge and now slice into cookie/size biscuits – remember they won't expand so the size and thickness you cut will be the size of the finished product.

Make the Chocolate topping

1: Melt the chocolate on the microwave for 1 min stir until smooth.

2: Add the butter – mix

Assemble the mint slices

1: Spread the biscuits with the peppermint cream.

2: Then pour on the chocolate topping.

3: Allow the chocolate to set

Nutrition Facts	Amount	% Daily Value*	Amount	% Daily Value*
	Total Fat 8.5g	13%	Total Carbohydrates 3g	1%
	Saturated 5.2g	26%	Dietary Fiber 1g	4%
Amount per 37 g	Trans Fat 0g		Sugars 0g	
1 serving (1.3 oz)	Cholesterol 49mg	16%	Protein 3g	5%
Calories 90	Sodium 56mg	2%		
From fat 75	Calcium 2% • Iron 5%		Vitamin A 5% • Vitamin C 0%	

HappyForks.com

* Percent Daily Values are based on 2000 calorie diet. Your Daily Values may be higher or lower depending on your calorie needs.

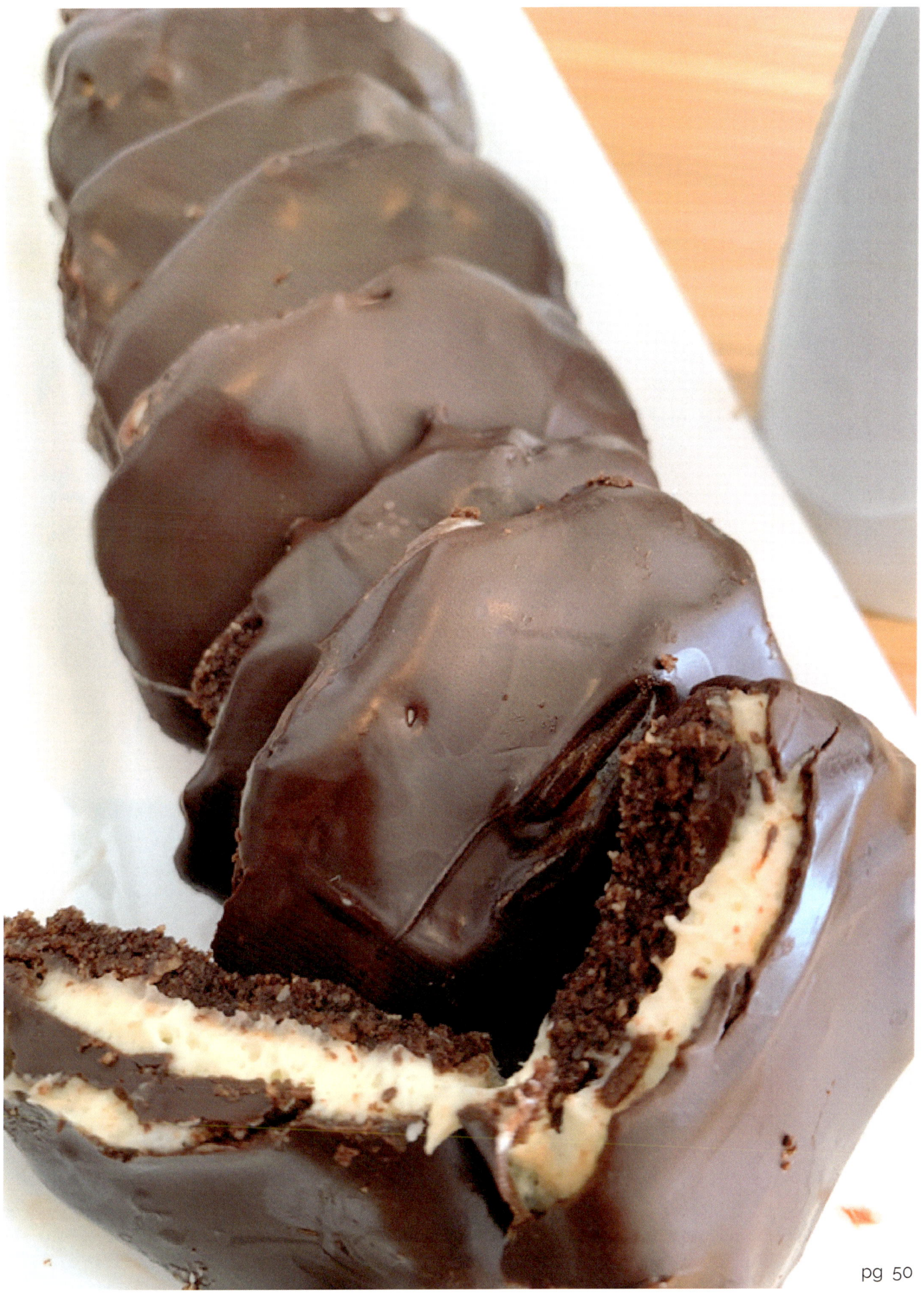

Viennese Fingers

Yield: Serves - 20 biscuits

Ingredients

1 cup Softened butter
6 Tbsp Powdered stevia
1 tsps. Vanilla essence
½ tsps. Salt
2 cups Coconut flour
4 Tbsp Rice flour
50g Suga- free dark chocolate

DIRECTIONS

1: Preheat oven 180°C.

2: Lightly grease 2 baking trays.

3: Beat the butter, sugar, vanilla essence, and salt in a mixing bowl until light and fluffy.

4: Gradually mix in the sifted coconut flour and rice flour.

5: Place the mixture in a piping bag fitted with a large star nozzle and pipe fingers about 5 cm long or in a circle on the baking tray allow for spreading.

6: in oven 12-15 minutes.

7: Leave to cool completely.

8: chocolate and dip ends to coat.

Nutrition Facts

Amount per 1 serving (0.6 oz): 16 g
Calories: 85
From fat: 69

Amount	% Daily Value*
Total Fat 7.8g	12%
Saturated 4.9g	25%
Trans Fat 0.3g	
Cholesterol 20mg	7%
Sodium 133mg	6%
Calcium 1% • Iron	5%

Amount	% Daily Value*
Total Carbohydrates 4g	1%
Dietary Fiber 0g	2%
Sugars 0g	
Protein 1g	1%
Vitamin A 7% • Vitamin C	3%

*Percent Daily Values are based on 2000 calorie diet. Your Daily Values may be higher or lower depending on your calorie needs.

HappyForks.com

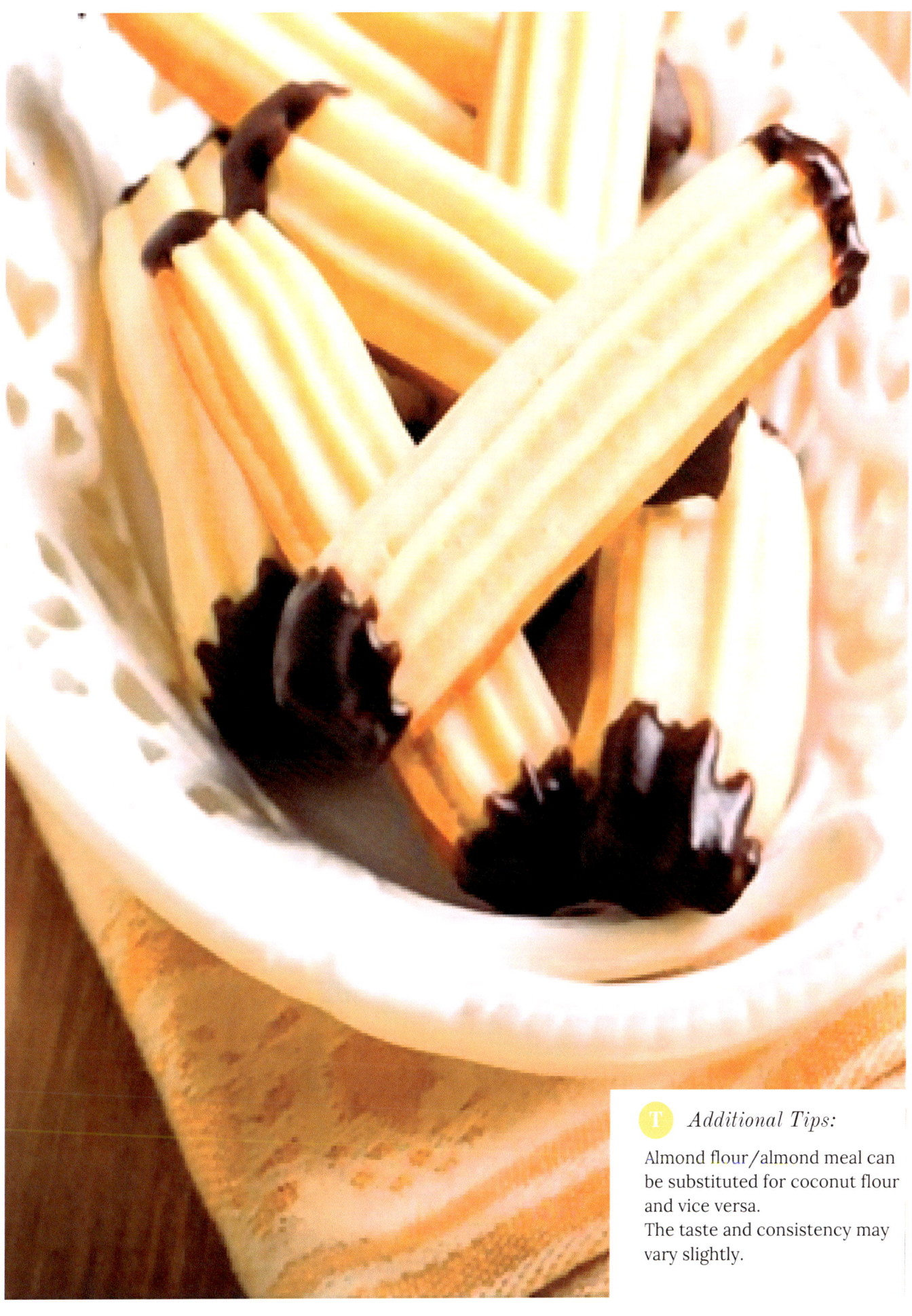

T *Additional Tips:*

Almond flour/almond meal can be substituted for coconut flour and vice versa.
The taste and consistency may vary slightly.

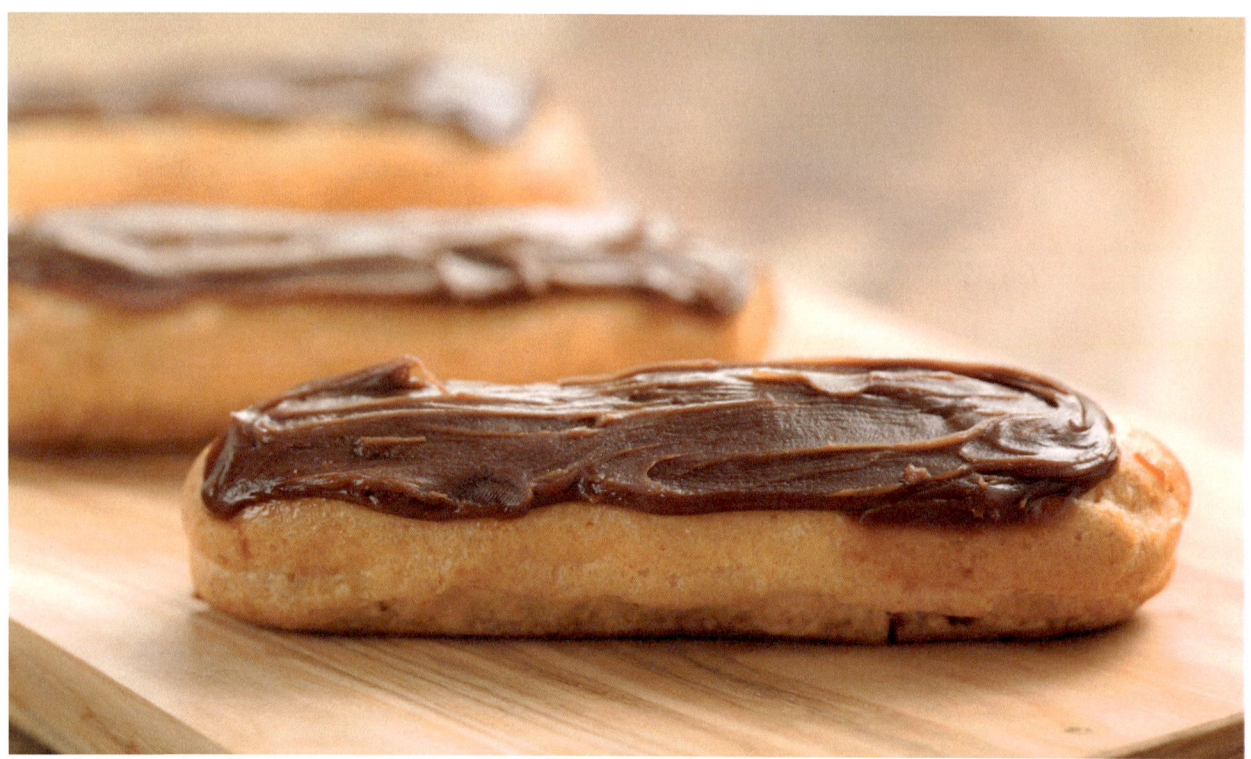

Éclairs

Ingredients

Yield: Makes approx. 30 mini or 15 large eclairs

('Choux') Pastry Ingredients

150ml Heavy cream
200ml Water
1 Cup Almond flour
3 Tbsp Coconut flour
1 Tbsp Psyllium powder
1 Tbsp Stevia
4 Medium eggs (*free-range*)
1 Large egg white-(*organic free-range*)
100g Butter (*grass-fed*)
1 Pinch sea salt
1 tsps. Baking powder

Filling Ingredients

½ cup Greek style yoghurt
100ml Heavy whipping cream
2 Tbsp Vanilla extract
1 coating Cinnamon
1 tsps. Ground clove
1 Tbsp Stevia

Glaze Ingredients

2 Tbsp Cacao powder
1 Tbsp Coconut oil
50g Butter grass-fed
1 Tbsp Stevia

Éclairs

DIRECTIONS

1. Preheat the oven to 200°C

2. Put the water, cream, butter, salt and sweetener in a large saucepan, and heat gently until the butter melts.

3. Remove from the heat and add the Psyllium husk powder, almond and coconut flour. Add the baking powder. Mix well to prevent any lumps from forming.

4. Return to the stove at low heat and mix with a wooden spoon or heat-resistant spatula until the mixture forms a dough that leaves the side of the pan clean.

5. Remove from the stove and let it cool for a few minutes. Gradually add eggs (one by one), beating well between each addition with a whisk. The dough needs to be smooth and glossy. (keep the egg white for later)

6. Line a large tray with baking paper and put the dough into a pastry bag and pipe out 10 cm long finger shaped eclairs.(allow space for rising, approx 2 cm)

7. Glaze them with the egg white and bake for 20 minutes. Leave them in the oven to cool down and don't open the oven.

8. While the Éclairs are cooling down, whip the cream and add vanilla, spices and sweetener. When the cream is firm, add in the greek yoghurt and mix well.

9. When the pastry is cooled, fill the piping bag with the cream and pipe in the filling until full. Put into the freezer for at least 20 minutes.

10. Place all the ingredients for the icing in a saucepan and heat them over medium temperature until they combine and form a smooth chocolate texture.

11. Pour the icing on cold Éclairs.

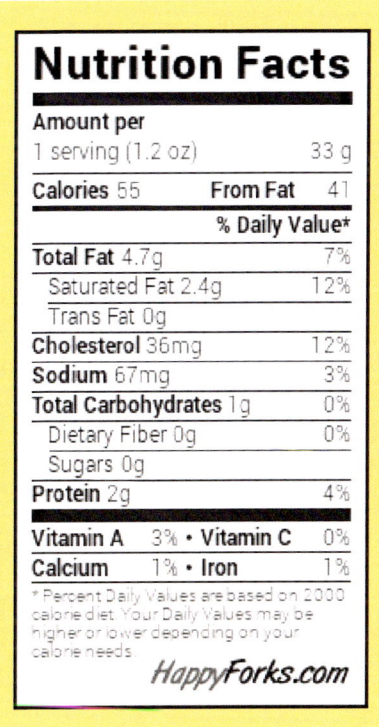

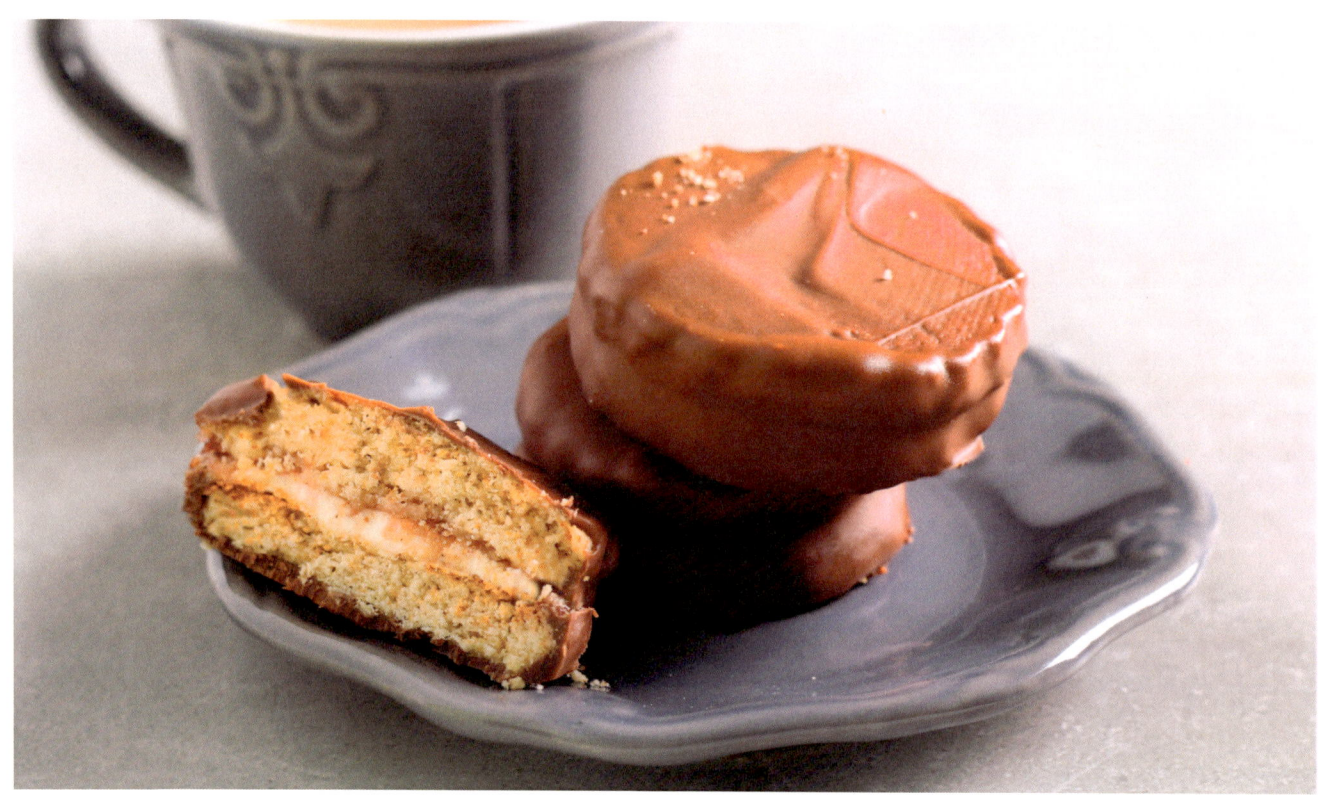

Pitch Your 'Wagon Wheels'

Ingredients

Yield: Servings 30

Biscuit

- 310g Peanut butter (*unsweetened*)
- 140g Stevia (*finely ground*)
- 2 Eggs (*Organic free-range*)
- 20g Cocoa powder (*organic*)
- 55g Blackberries (*frozen is fine*)
- 25g Butter (*kerry gold*)
- 35g Gelatine powder
- 2 tsps. Vanilla extract
- 1 tsps. Cinnamon powder
- 10g Baking powder
- Pinch pink Himalayan salt

Marshmallow layer

- 25g Sugar free icing sugar (Sukrin)
- 100ml water
- 25g Gelatine powder
- ¼ tsp Vanilla extract

Assembly

- 150g sugar-free raspberry jam *
- 100g Sugar free dark chocolate

* use *Amarenta* recipe from black forest cake recipe and substitute raspberries for the cherries to make your jam.

Pitch Your 'Wagon Wheels'

Biscuit Method

1. Preheat oven to 170 °C. Line 2 large baking trays with baking paper.

2. Combine all biscuit ingredients in a large bowl or mixer until well combined.

3. Roll out cookie dough between two sheets of baking paper until 1-2mm thickness. Using a 5 cm cookie cutter, cut into 60 biscuits and place in single layer on baking trays.

4. Bake 7 minutes or until the edges of the cookies are just starting to brown or feel crisp.

5. Cool on wire rack whilst you work on the rest of the recipe.

Marshmallow Method

1. In a small saucepan, over medium heat dissolve stevia in half of the water.

2. Add gelatin to remaining water and stir to combine. Add to saucepan and whisk to dissolve.

Assembly Method:

1. Spread 30 biscuits with 1 teaspoon of sugar free jam and top with a spoon full of marshmallow. Sandwich with another biscuit and gently squish marshmallow to spread. Place onto tray and refrigerate until set.

2. Melt the sugar free chocolate in the microwave or on baine-marie.
Coat the biscuits with the chocolate.
Refrigerate until set.

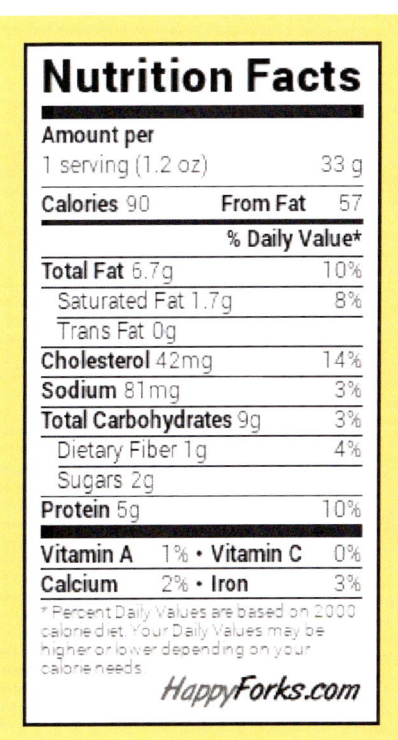

Venus Bars (Not from 'Mars')

This creation will absolutely fool you that it is NOT sugar. Sukrin:1 is erythritol, which is a polyol. Polyols are carbohydrates that have **no effect on blood sugar**.
With the addition of the protein to make the soft nougat centre it would also substitute as a great protein snack bar. Either way it's an absolute winner.

Serves 12

Ingredients

Chocolate Nougat
180g Sukrin Clear Fibre Syrup
20g Sugar-Free dark chocolate
130g Whey protein isolate
1 Tbsp M.C.T Oil
(Medium Chain Triglycerides -clear oil made from coconut)

Caramel
200g Sukrin Gold Fibre Syrup
60g Butter
80g Thickened cream

Coating
140g Sugar-Free Milk Chocolate

DIRECTIONS

1: Place clear syrup and chocolate in large heat proof bowl and microwave for 1 minute. Stir to combine until smooth.

2: Combine chocolate mix with protein powder and MCT oil and mix until combined

3: Allow the mix to cool at ambient temperature - it will start to thicken.

4: Spoon or break off pieces and push into moulds (will make 32 x 4cm moulds)

5: Allow the mix to cool at ambinet temperature - it will start to thicken. Let it cool while you prepare the caramel layer.

Nutrition Facts
Amount per 1 serving (2.4 oz) 69 g
Calories 108   From Fat 60
% Daily Value*
Total Fat 6.9g — 11%
 Saturated Fat 3.7g — 18%
 Trans Fat 0.2g
Cholesterol 16mg — 5%
Sodium 92mg — 4%
Total Carbohydrates 4g — 1%
 Dietary Fiber 1g — 5%
 Sugars 1g
Protein 11g — 21%
Vitamin A 6% • Vitamin C 4%
Calcium 4% • Iron 10%
* Percent Daily Values are based on a 2000 calorie diet. Your Daily Values may be higher or lower depending on your calorie needs.

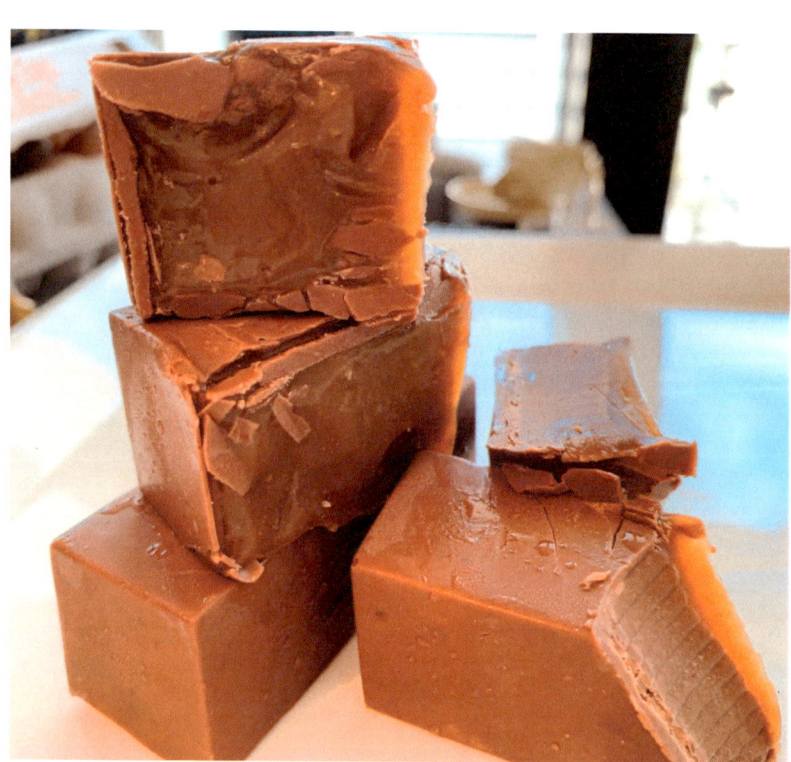

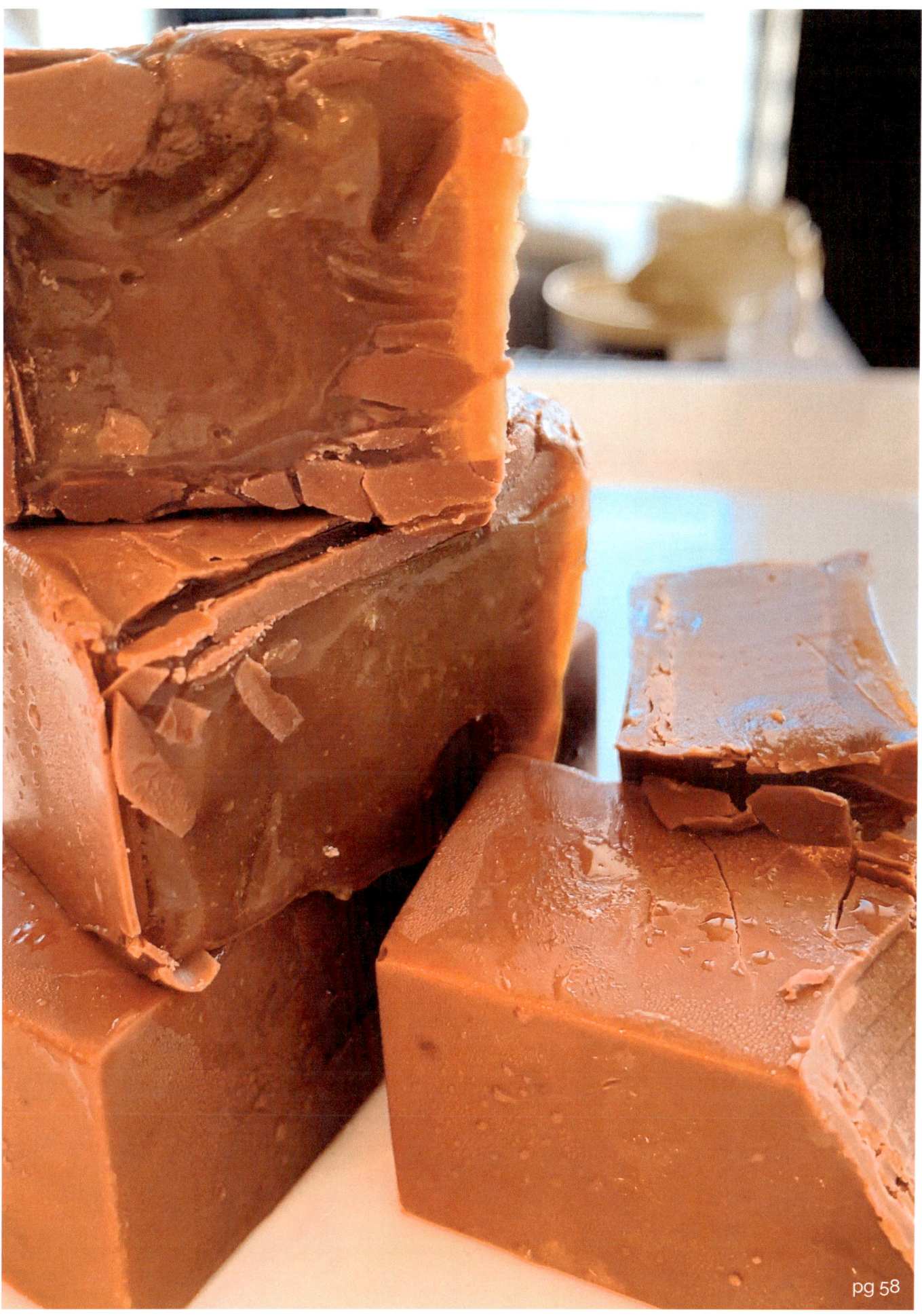

pg 58

Venus Bars (Not from 'Mars')

Take your time with this recipe as it needs to be made in stages and allowed to cool. It's best to put the silicon chocolate mould in the freezer. Then when you have melted the sugar free chocolate spread it around the mould. Let the chocolate set in the freezer for a few minutes and then began to 'build' your *mars* bar.

First make the nougat and when it's smooth and well blended place it inside the chocolate lined moulds. Allow this layer to set. Now you are ready to prepare the caramel layer.

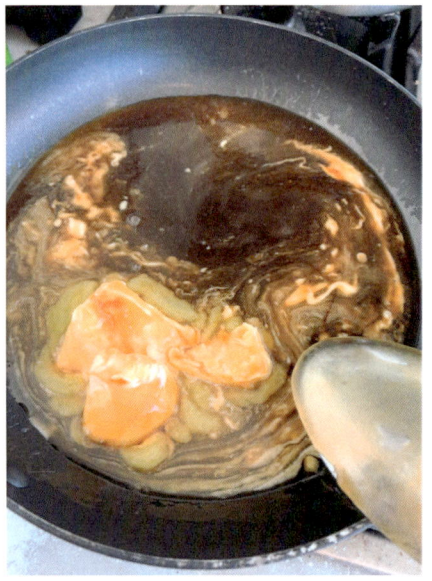 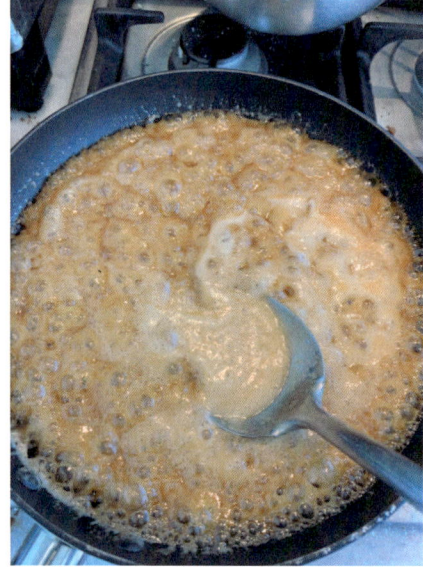 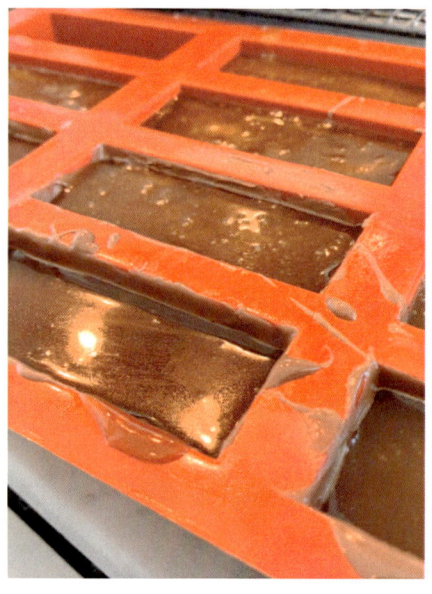

Step 1:

Place all caramel ingredients into a non-stick heavy based pan.

Step 2:

Heat on high until the butter melts and the mixture starts to bubble. The mixture will become thicker and more viscose. At this point you will definitely smell that beautiful caramel scent.

Step 3:

Carefully spoon the hot caramel into your moulds. Refrigerate until set.

Melt chocolate and add the final top coat to each '*mars bar*'.

After you have finished the top coat of chocolate. Allow this to cool again. Place back in the freezer for a few minutes.

Now you are ready to pop out your keto mars bars and enjoy!

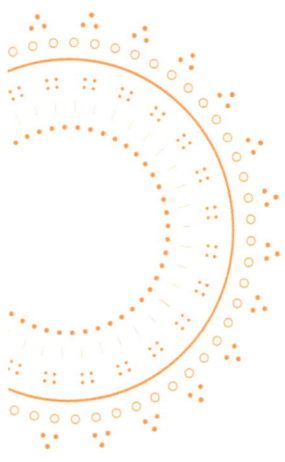

White Chocolate - Sugar Free

Serves 12

Ingredients

75 g Cocoa butter
3 Tbsp Coconut oil
¼ tsp Liquid sunflower lecithin
¼ cup Finely Powdered stevia
¼ cup Heavy cream powder
(*or whole milk powder*)
½ tsp Vanilla Extract
1/16 tsp Sea salt (*optional*)

DIRECTIONS

1: Cut the cocoa butter into small pieces, no larger than 1/2 in (1.3 cm) in any direction. This important to prevent overheating the outside when melting.

2: Place the cocoa butter, coconut oil, and sunflower lecithin into a small saucepan. Melt on the stove over VERY low heat. Do not allow it to simmer or boil. (Even better, use a double boiler if you can.) Remove from heat once melted.

3: Stir in the sweetener, until dissolved. Stir in the cream powder, vanilla extract, and sea salt, until smooth.

4: Pour into chocolate molds (or onto a small baking paper lined pan). Refrigerate until hardened. Keep refrigerated for best results.

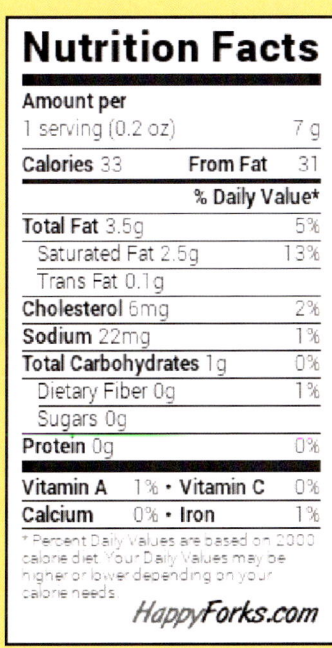

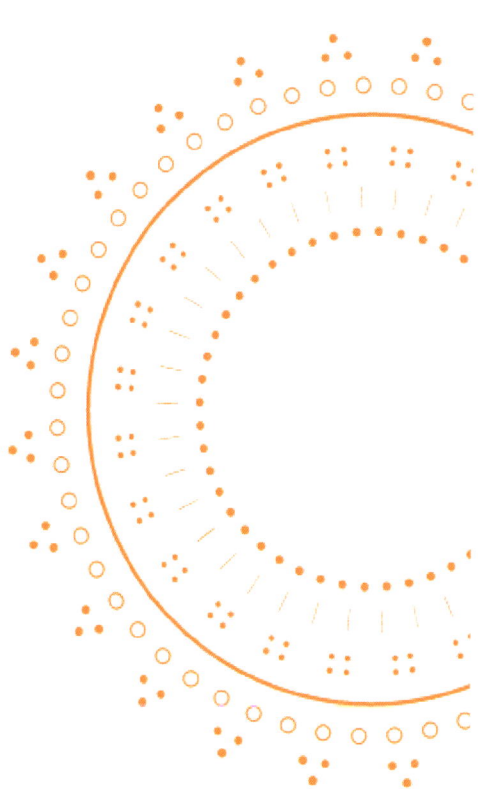

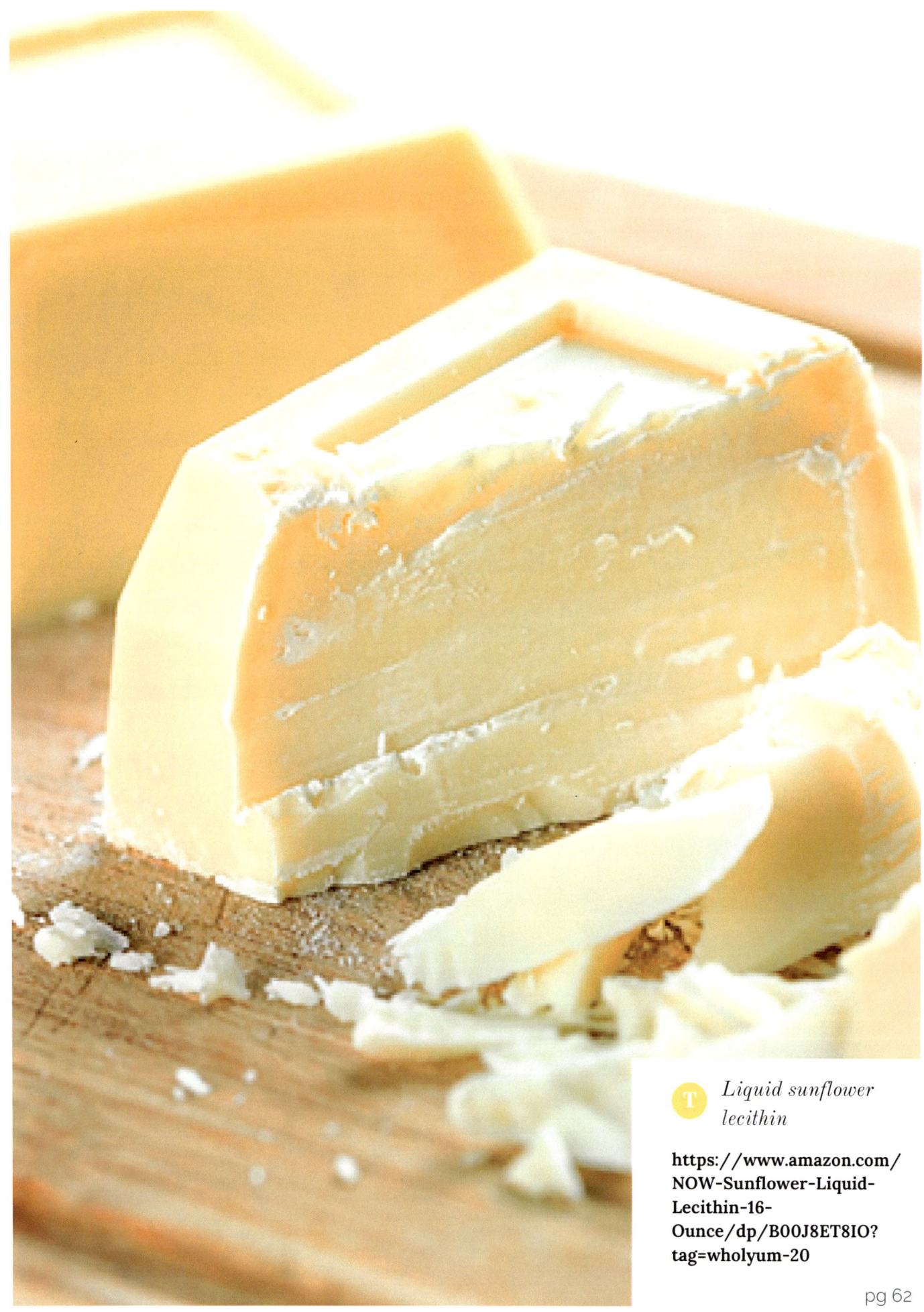

T Liquid sunflower lecithin

https://www.amazon.com/NOW-Sunflower-Liquid-Lecithin-16-Ounce/dp/B00J8ET8IO?tag=wholyum-20

'Snackers' Bar

Yield: 12 large bars

Ingredients

'Cream' Layer:
⅓ cup Cashews, soaked, unsalted (*weighed before soaking*)
1 ½ Tbsp Coconut cream
1 ½ Tbsp Sukrin Gold fibre syrup
½ tsps. Sugar-free vanilla extract

Caramel Layer:
3 tbsp All natural peanut butter (*no sugar added*)
2 tsp (10ml) Sukrin clear fibre syrup
1 tbsp Granulated Stevia
2 tbsp Melted butter
handful whole peanuts

Chocolate Layer:
50g Sugar-free chocolate
75g Additional chocolate for topcoat

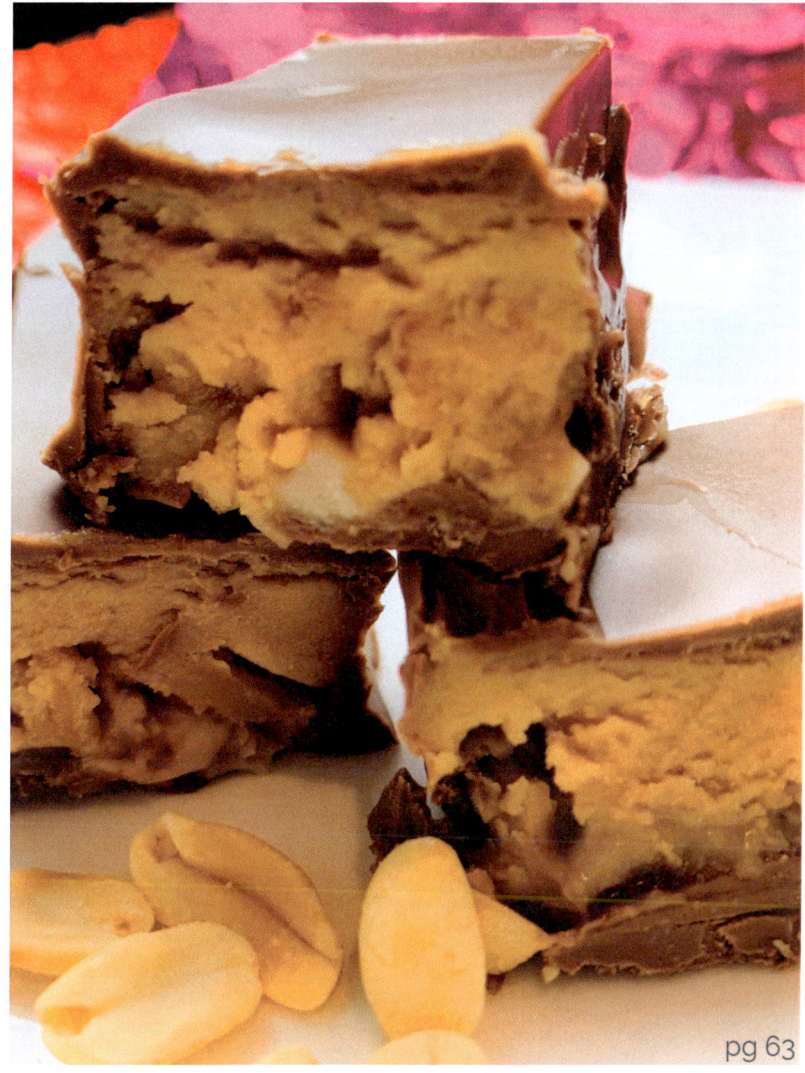

Nutrition Facts

Amount per 1 serving (0.9 oz) 25 g

Calories 75	From Fat 52	
		% Daily Value*
Total Fat 6.1g		9%
Saturated Fat 2.7g		14%
Trans Fat 0.1g		
Cholesterol 5mg		2%
Sodium 76mg		3%
Total Carbohydrates 5g		2%
Dietary Fiber 1g		4%
Sugars 2g		
Protein 2g		4%
Vitamin A 1%	• Vitamin C	0%
Calcium 0%	• Iron	2%

* Percent Daily Values are based on 2000 calorie diet. Your Daily Values may be higher or lower depending on your calorie needs

'Snackers' Bar

Method:

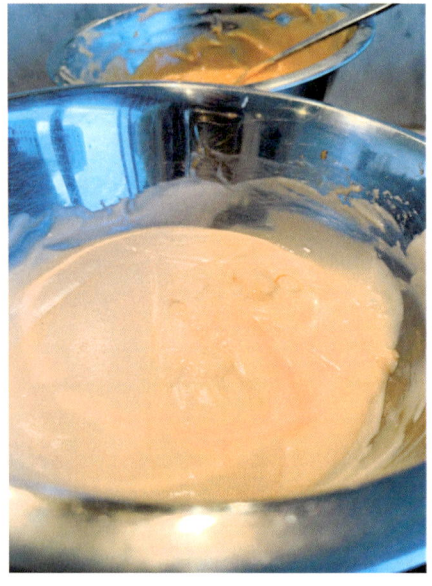
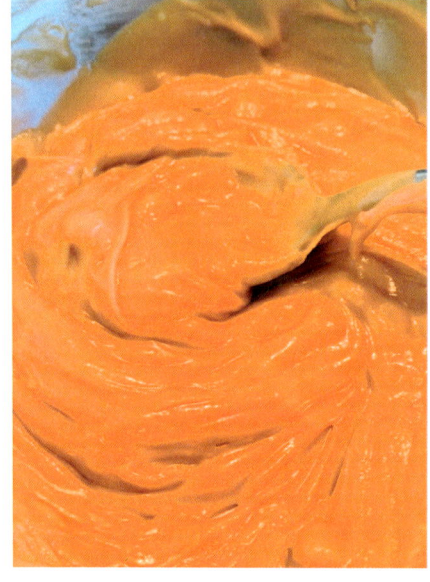
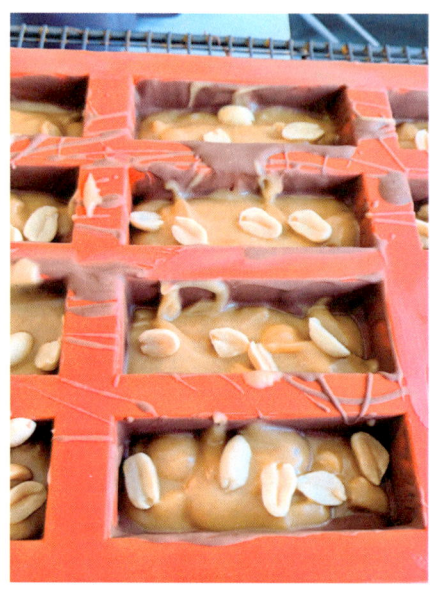

Cream Layer

1. Add the ingredients for the "*cream*" layer (soaked cashews, coconut cream, gold fibre syrup & vanilla extract) into a food processor and blend for at least 1-2 minutes until you get a smooth and chunk-free, cream-like mass.

2. Chill in the fridge while you continue to the next step.

Chocolate base

1. Melt the sugar-free chocolate in the microwave or use a double boiler.

2. Pour the chocolate into rectangular shaped silicone molds. The bottom of the mold should be fully covered but don't add too much chocolate (about 5mm is enough).

3. Place the mold with the chocolate into your freezer for approx. 10 minutes until the chocolate has hardened.

4. Add the cashew cream into the silicone mold as well. Press the creme into shape using your fingers.

5. Place back in your freezer for approx. 15 minutes while you prepare the "caramel" layer.

Caramel Layer

1. In a large mixing bowl add the sukrin fibre syrup, peanut butter and stevia except for the whole the peanuts.

2. Melt the butter in the microwave.

3. Add the melted butter to the rest of the caramel layer. Mix together until smooth.

Assembly

1. Pour the caramel layer on top of the cream layer into the silicone mold.

2. Place the whole peanuts on top of the caramel layer and chill again for 15 minutes in your freezer before popping the bars out of the silicone mold.

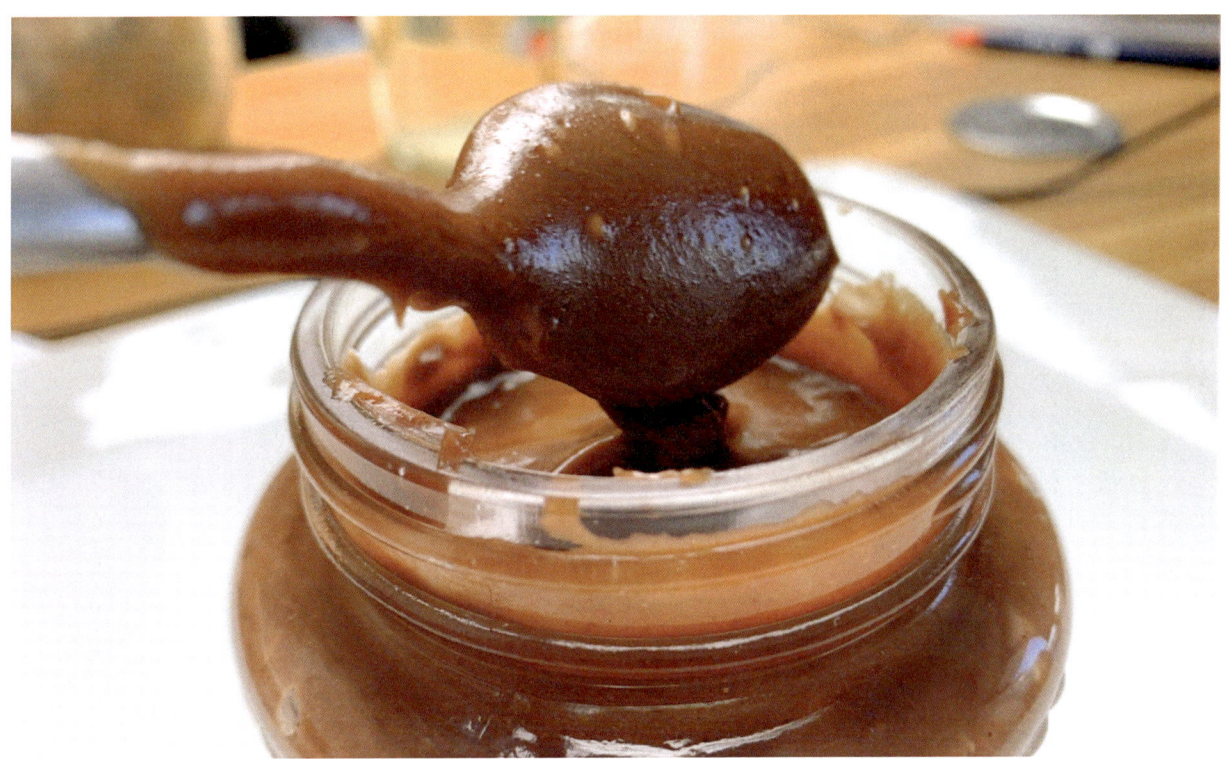

Chocolate Hazelnut Spread A.k.a 'Nutella'

Ingredients:

Yield: 500 g or 2 cups

1 cup Peeled hazelnuts
1 cup Macadamia nuts
½ cup Almonds
100 g Sugar-free dark chocolate
1 tbsp Virgin coconut oil
2 tsps. Liquid Stevia
1 Tbsp Cacao powder
1-2 tsps. Vanilla extract
120 ml Coconut milk
(*or heavy whipping cream*)

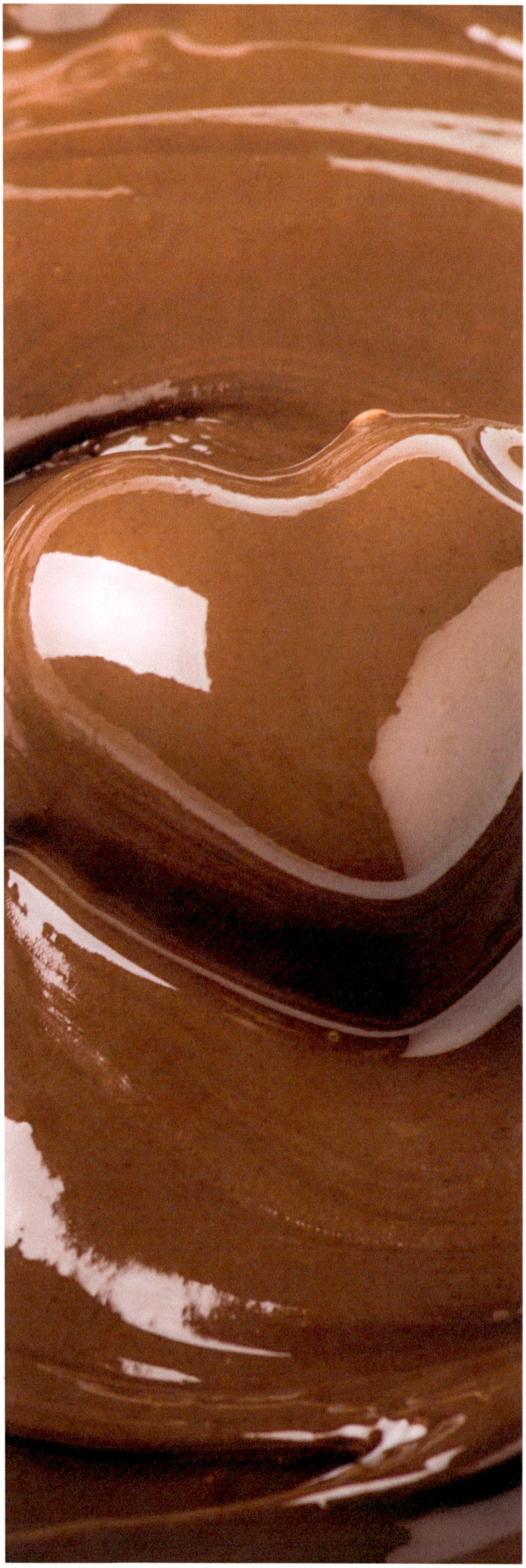

1. Preheat the oven to 190 °C. Spread the hazelnuts, macadamia nuts, and almonds on a baking tray and transfer to the oven. Bake for about 8-10 minutes, until lightly browned. Remove the nuts from the oven and let them cool for 15 minutes.

2. Melt the chocolate in the microwave in a heat proof container for approx. 1 min. Alternatively use a double boiler.

3. Place the nuts into a food processor and pulse until smooth.

4. Add the melted chocolate, coconut oil, liquid stevia, cacao powder and vanilla powder. Pulse until smooth. If you're using coconut milk, slowly drizzle it to the processor while blending (to prevent the chocolate from splitting, use <u>warm coconut milk or cream</u> the <u>same temperature</u> as the warm chocolate.

5. Pour into a jar and let it cool down and refrigerate for up to 3 months (or up to 1 week if you're using cream or coconut milk)

Enjoy any way you would love your *'Nutella!'*

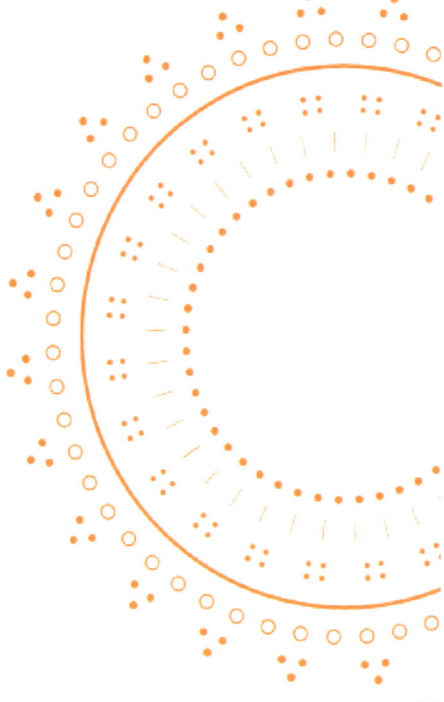

'Pop Your 'Cherry Ripe' Bars

Yield: Makes approx. 12 bars

Ingredients

2 cups Desiccated coconut
3 Tbsp Coconut oil
3 Tbsp 'no-sugar' fibre syrup (*like sukritol*)
1 tsps. Vanilla extract
1 cup "Amarenta" (*cherry jam*) *see recipe

Chocolate coating
300 grams 'no-sugar' dark chocolate, (*melted*)

*Amarenta (cherry jam)
375 g pitted cherries (*Fresh or frozen*)
8 tsps. Liquid stevia
¾ cup water
2 Tbsp Ground chia seeds

DIRECTIONS

1: Prep: Start by making the Amarenta (cherry jam)

Method : Amarenta

If using fresh cherries Wash the cherries and remove the pits. Or you may use frozen pitted cherries. Add them to a heavy based stainless steel pan.

2: Add the stevia, 3/4 cup of water and 2 tablespoons of chia seeds

3: Place on a stove and cook over low-medium heat. Slowly bring to a boil and mix frequently until the juices slightly thicken. This may take 20-30 minutes. When done, your amarenata should be thickened into a syrup and the flavour very strong - just like sweet cherry extract. It will thicken even more when chilled.

Nutrition Facts

Amount per 45 g
1 serving (1.6 oz)
Calories 107
From fat 47

	Amount	% Daily Value*		Amount	% Daily Value*
Total Fat	5.5g	9%	Total Carbohydrates	14g	5%
Saturated	4.3g	22%	Dietary Fiber	2g	7%
Trans Fat	0g		Sugars	9g	
Cholesterol	0mg	0%	Protein	1g	3%
Sodium	77mg	3%			
Calcium	9% • Iron	3%	Vitamin A	1% • Vitamin C	8%

*Percent Daily Values are based on 2000 calorie diet. Your Daily Values may be higher or lower depending on your calorie needs.

HappyForks.com

'Pop Your 'Cherry Ripe' Bars

Chocolate Method:

1. Line a square 20cm tin with baking paper over-hanging the sides for easy removal.

2. Divide chocolate into thirds - Break chocolate into pieces and place in a heat proof microwave jug.

3. Cook on high for one minute until chocolate is runny.

4. Blend chocolate into the coconut oil and mix well.

5. Pour into lined tin. Smooth with a spatula. Place in the freezer to set.

Cherry Coconut filling:

1. Place 1 cup of the desiccated coconut, the coconut oil, sugar-free syrup and vanilla to your processor and blend at high speed until the mixture is well combined and the coconut has broken down. Spoon the mixture into a bowl and set aside.

2. Place the cherry jam and the remaining 1 cup of desiccated coconut into your processor and blend at high speed until the mixture is broken down and well combined. Add the coconut mixture to the cherry mixture and blend at high speed to combine.

3. Press the mixture firmly into your tin and place in the freezer for 20 min to set.

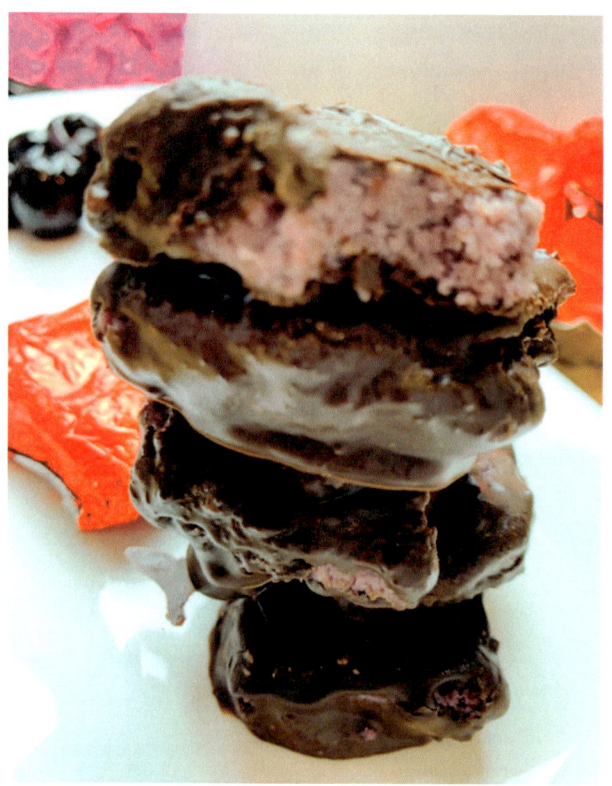

Top layer of chocolate:

1. Melt more chocolate and cover the filling - smoothing with a spatula.

2. Place again in the freezer for 20 min to set.

3. Once set, cut them into squares.

Double Coating Chocolate

1. Melt the final third of chocolate.

2. Use two forks to dip the *cherry ripes* coating them with the melted chocolate. Once coated sit them on a tray lined with baking paper and return to the fridge.

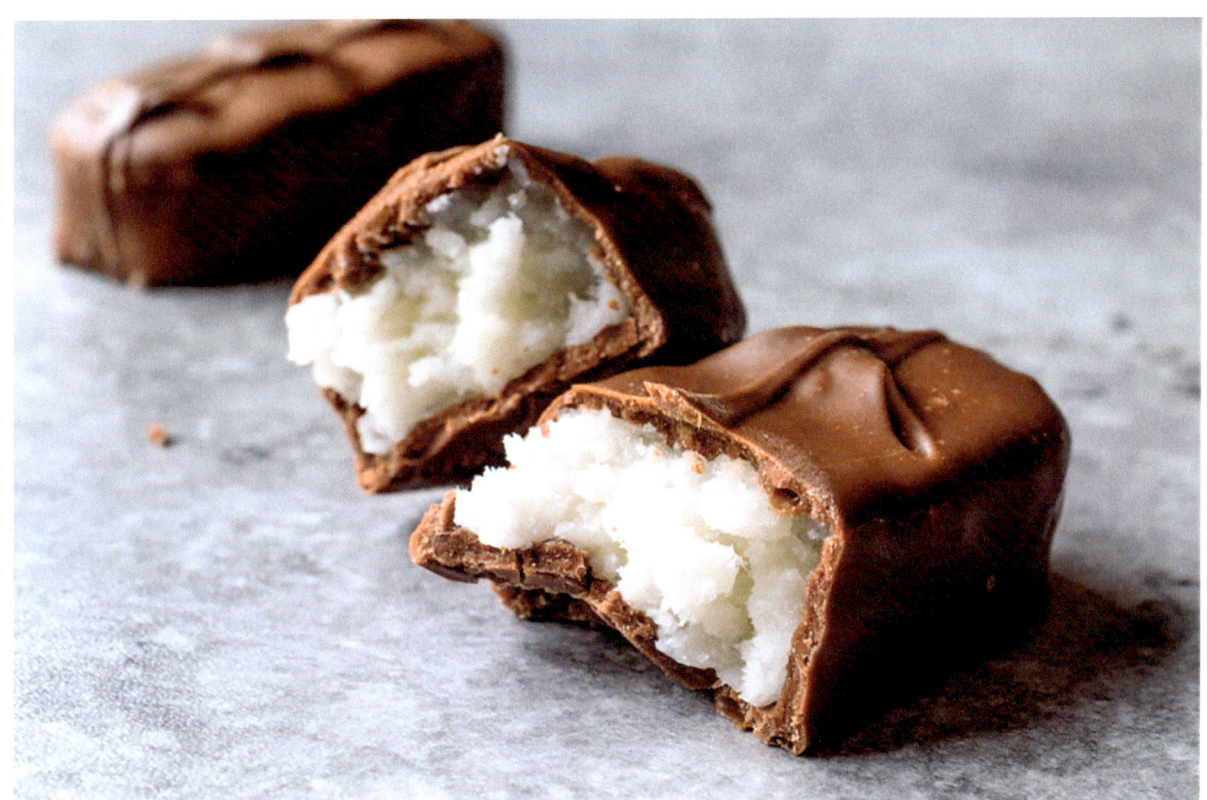

Mutiny on the 'Bounty' Bars

Ingredients

Chocolate coating
300g sugar-free milk chocolate

Sugar Free 'Condensed Milk' Recipe
300 ml heavy cream
2 tablespoons butter (*melted*)
2/3 cup powdered stevia
1 tsps. smooth peanut butter
½ tsps. vanilla extract

Filling
2½ cups desiccated coconut
½ cup stevia powdered (*finely blended*)
¼ tsps. vanilla
¾ cup condensed milk

Mutiny on the 'Bounty' Bars

Method

'Condensed milk'

1. Place all the ingredients together in a heavy based pot.

2. Simmer on a low -medium heat until you achieve a very thick consistency akin to condensed milk or a heavy custard. (coats the back of a spoon)

Chocolate coating

1. Place approx. 200g of the milk chocolate in a microwave for approximately one minute or until melted and mixes smoothly.

2. Line a silicone mould with sugar free milk chocolate.

3. Tip the melted chocolate all around the sides so that mould is evenly coated. Set the chocolate in the freezer for a few minutes to harden.

Prepare the filling.

1. Put the powdered stevia in a powerful blender or coffee grinder to make a fine "icing sugar" consistency.

2. Add the desiccated coconut and stevia together.

3. Then add the vanilla and *condensed milk* mix.

Assemble

1. Add the filling in to the chocolate lined moulds.

2. Place in the fridge to set.

Chocolate coating

1. Place approx. 100g of the milk chocolate in a microwave for approximately one minute or until melted and mixes smoothly.

2. When the filling has set pour a top layer over the filling.

3. Place in the freezer for 2-3 minutes to set the chocolate quickly.

4. Remove from the freezer - unmould. drizzle some more chocolate on the top for an extra thick chocolate layer and give it that authentic bounty design.

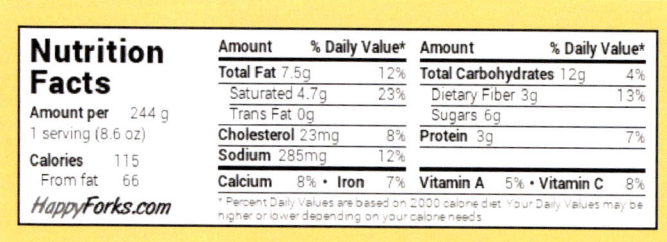

'Twax' Bars
Yield: approximately 30 biscuits

Ingredients:

Biscuit Ingredients
12 Tbsp   Butter
50g Cream cheese
1   Egg
1 Cup   Sulkrin powdered sugar-free icing sugar
½ tsps.   Liquid Stevia
1 tsps. Pink Himalayan salt
1 tsps. Almond extract
¼ tsps.   Xantham gum
2 Cups   Almond flour
½ Cup Coconut flour

Caramel Ingredients
100g   Butter
½ Cup Heavy Cream
2 Tbsp   Sukrin (sugar free) dark syrup
1 tsps. Vanilla Extract

Chocolate Ganache Ingredients
½ Cup Heavy Cream
½ Cup Sugar-Free Dark Chocolate

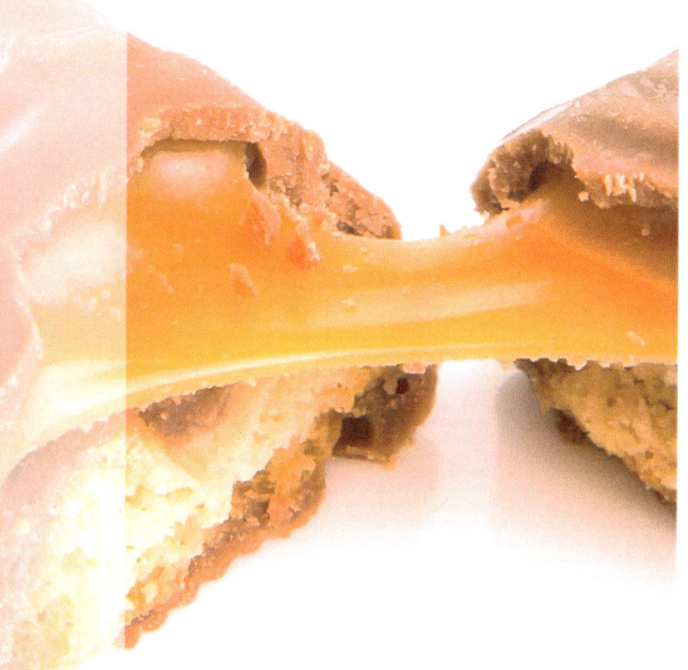

'Twax' Bars

Method

1. In a large mixing bowl add the cream, butter and cream cheese and beat with a hand mixer until smooth.

2. Add the egg, sukrin 'icing sugar', liquid stevia, salt, and vanilla. Beat until smooth.

3. Add the remaining dry ingredients and mix until well incorporated.

4. Let your biscuit dough rest for a minimum of 4 hours.

5. After your biscuit has rested remove from the fridge and dust your kitchen countertop with fine coconut flour.

6. Place your dough in between two baking sheets or silicone matts and roll until the dough is about 0.5 cm thick.

7. Remove the top baking sheet and use a cookie cutter to make cookie shapes. Alternatively, you can make into finger sized biscuits like the real "*twix*"

8. Bake the cookies for about 10 mins at 170 degrees – The time and temperature will vary depending on your oven. (*See the back-oven temperature conversion chart to help you.*)

9. When the cookies are golden brown remove and allow to cool on a wire rack.

Prepare the caramel centre

1. In a heavy based pan heat the butter, sukrin syrup until it starts to bubble.

2. Slowly add the cream and vanilla, keep whisking as it bubbles. It should start to thicken and rise.

3. Remove your pan from the heat and continue to whisk until it stops bubbling.

4. Allow it to completely cool before you start to use it.

Prepare the chocolate ganache.

1. Heat up the cream in a saucepan.

2. Place the chocolate in a stainless-steel heatproof bowl.

3. When the cream comes just before the boil add to the chocolate and mix well until the chocolate completely melts and has a smooth consistency.

Assembly.

1. Take your biscuits and add a thick spoonful of the caramel.

2. Then coat with the chocolate ganache.

Nutrition Facts	Amount	% Daily Value*	Amount	% Daily Value*
Amount per 34 g 1 serving (1.2 oz)	Total Fat 7.6g	12%	Total Carbohydrates 8g	3%
	Saturated 4.6g	23%	Dietary Fiber 0g	1%
	Trans Fat 0g		Sugars 0g	
Calories 75	Cholesterol 38mg	13%	Protein 1g	2%
From fat 68	Sodium 75mg	3%		
HappyForks.com	Calcium 1% • Iron 2%		Vitamin A 5% • Vitamin C 0%	

*Percent Daily Values are based on 2000 calorie diet. Your Daily Values may be higher or lower depending on your calorie needs

Chocolate Mousse

Serves 12

Ingredients

2 Egg whites
300g Sugar-free dark chocolate
400ml Thickened cream

Optional:
1 Tbsp of liquid Stevia to sweeten, mixed with whipped cream

DIRECTIONS

1: In a medium, very dry mixing bowl place the egg whites and beat until soft peaks are formed. Set aside.

2: In a separate bowl, beat the cream with an electric mixture until it begins to thicken. Be careful not to overbeat.

3: Melt the sugar free dark chocolate until runny and smooth (either over a double-boiler or broken up in the microwave on high in 30 second batches, stirring in between).

4: While the chocolate is hot, begin to beat the cream and pour sugar free dark chocolate in at the same time until it's just mixed through.

5: Fold in the egg whites using a spatula.

6: Spoon or pipe the mousse into individual jars and refrigerate for at least 4 hours. Garnish with extra cream, mint or strawberries

Nutrition Facts

Amount per
1 serving (2.3 oz) — 64 g

Calories 129 — From Fat 113

% Daily Value*

- Total Fat 12.8g — 20%
- Saturated Fat 7.9g — 39%
- Trans Fat 0g
- Cholesterol 46mg — 15%
- Sodium 107mg — 4%
- Total Carbohydrates 5g — 2%
- Dietary Fiber 1g — 3%
- Sugars 1g
- Protein 2g — 4%

Vitamin A 10% • Vitamin C 0%
Calcium 2% • Iron 3%

* Percent Daily Values are based on 2000 calorie diet. Your Daily Values may be higher or lower depending on your calorie needs

HappyForks.com

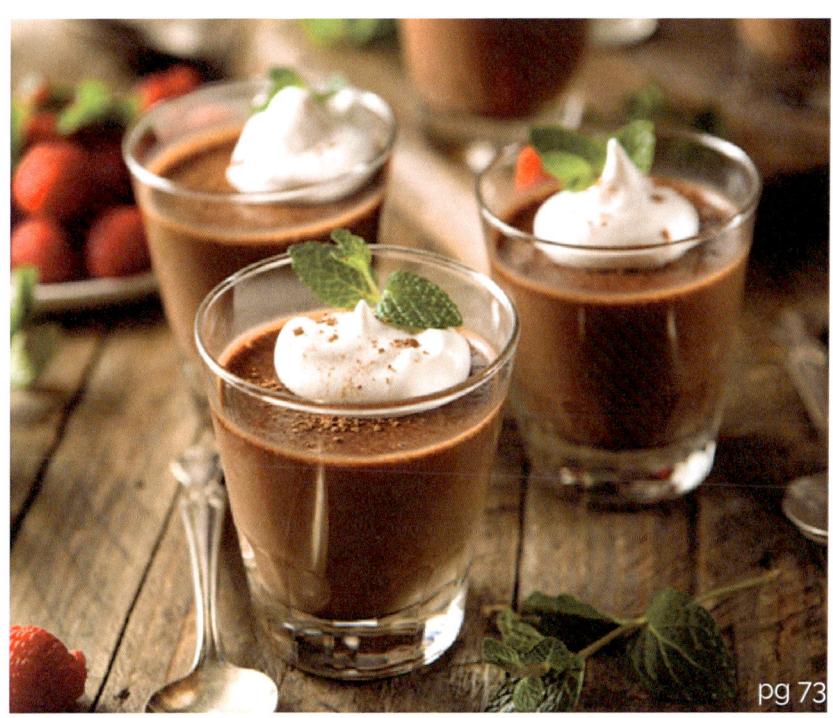

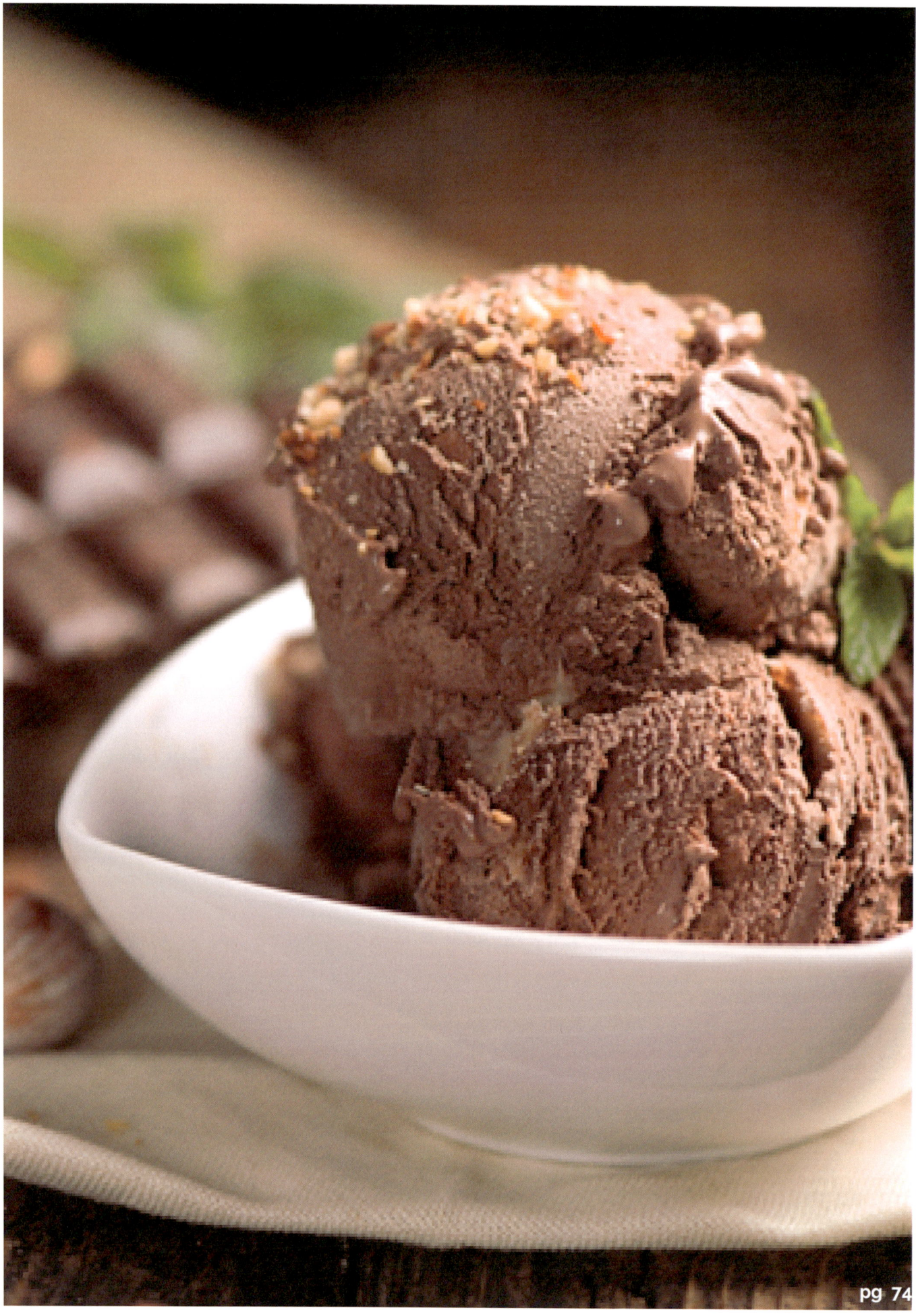

No-Sugar Chocolate Ice Cream

Ice cream is our favourite go to food to comfort us. So this recipe will keep that special soothing extravagance without feeling any guilt.

Serves 10

Ingredients

2 cups Heavy cream (*organic*)

1 cup Coconut milk (*organic*)

½ cup Cocoa powder (*unsweetened*)

6 Large egg yolks (*organic free-range*)

2/3 cup Stevia -powdered

1/8 tsps. Vanilla extract

1/16 tsps. Pink Sea salt

¼ tsps. Xanthan gum

200g Sugar-free dark chocolate

DIRECTIONS

1: Grind stevia/xylitol in a blender/coffee grinder to make a very fine powder.

2: In a small saucepan, simmer heavy cream, coconut milk, sifted cocoa powder, stevia, vanilla, xanthan gum and salt until the powdered stevia completely dissolves, about 5 minutes. Remove pan from heat.

3: In a separate bowl, whisk egg yolks.

4: Whisking constantly, slowly pour about one-third of the hot cream into the yolks, then whisk the yolk mixture back into the pot of cream.

5: Return pan to medium-low heat and gently cook until mixture is thick enough to coat the back of a spoon

6: Cool mixture to room temperature. Cover and chill overnight in the refrigerator.

7: Melt the sugar free dark chocolate either over a double boiler or in the microwave. Fold into the cream mix. For an added texture you can reserve some of the chocolate and just roughly chop and mix through.

8: Churn liquid in an ice-cream machine. Serve directly from the machine for soft serve, or store in freezer until needed.

Nutrition Facts

Amount per 1 serving (3.1 oz) — 88 g

Calories 150	From Fat 118

	% Daily Value*
Total Fat 13.4g	21%
Saturated Fat 7.5g	37%
Trans Fat 0g	
Cholesterol 146mg	49%
Sodium 110mg	5%
Total Carbohydrates 13g	4%
Dietary Fiber 2g	9%
Sugars 2g	
Protein 4g	9%
Vitamin A 11% • Vitamin C	0%
Calcium 6% • Iron	7%

† Percent Daily Values are based on 2000 calorie diet. Your Daily values may be higher or lower depending on your calorie needs.

HappyForks.com

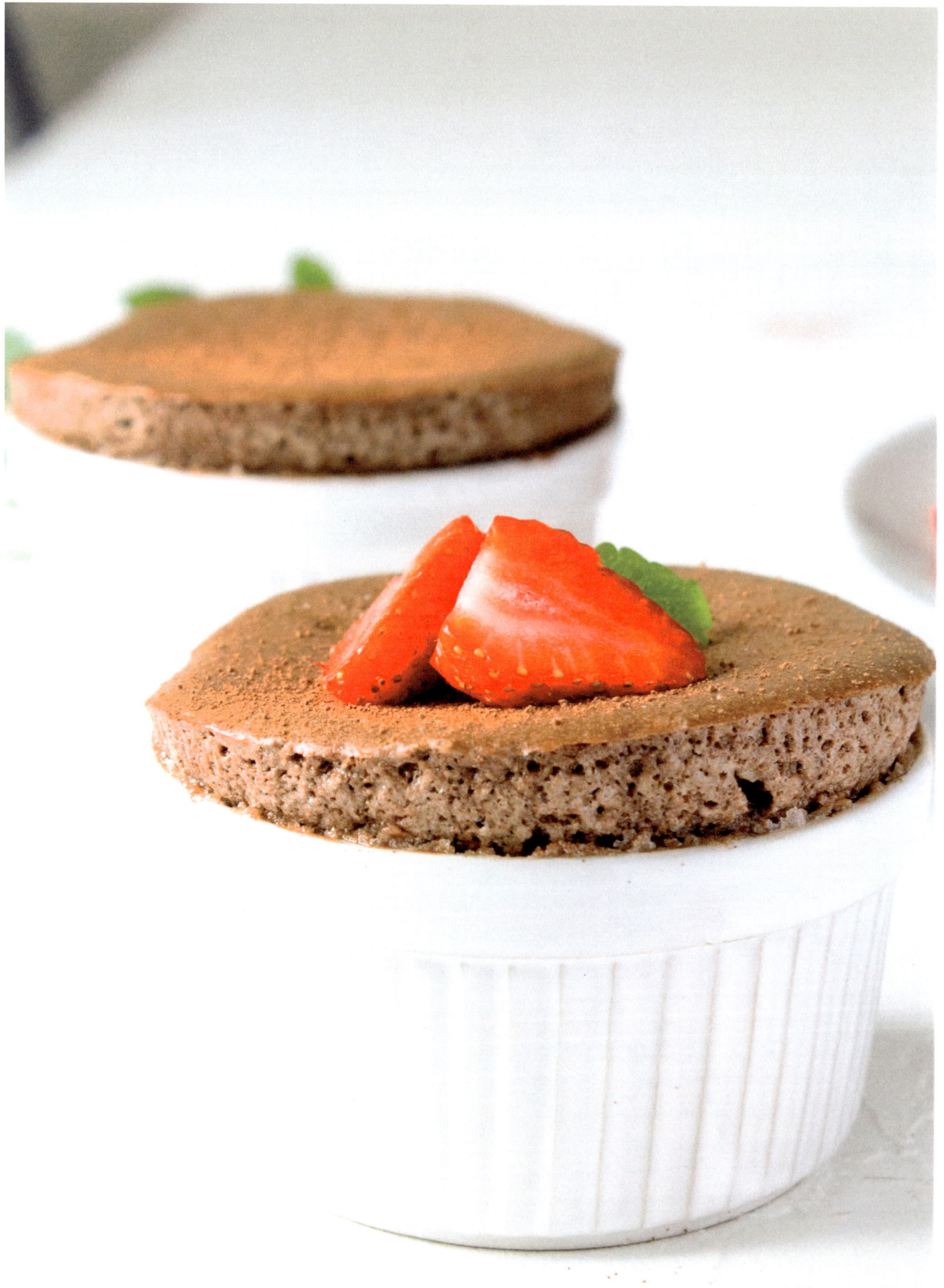

Chocolate Souffle

Yield: Serves 4 x 1 cup sized ramekins

Ingredients

5 large eggs (*separated*)
125g Sugar-free dark chocolate
1 Tbsp Coconut oil
1 Tbsp Butter
(*for greasing ramekins*)
¼ tsps. Cream of tartar
Pinch of pink Himalayan salt
4 Tbsp powdered stevia
(*Plus 1 Tbsp for 'flouring'*)
1 tsps. Cacao powder
1 tsps. Vanilla extract

Optional:

Sugar free icing sugar
Whipped cream

DIRECTIONS

1: Preheat your oven to 190C. Prepare four 1 cup sized ramekins by greasing with butter and "*flouring*" with 1 Tbsp of the powdered stevia. Set aside.

2: Place the chocolate and coconut oil in a microwave safe bowl and melt for approximately 1 minute in 30 sec batches stirring occasionally. Ensure the oil and chocolate mix smoothly together. Leave to cool.

3: Separate egg yolks and whites into 2 separate mixing bowls.

4: Beat the egg whites using an electric whisk until stiff peaks form. As they start to froth add the cream of tartar, salt and half the powdered stevia.

5: Beat the egg yolks with the rest of sweetener until pale in colour. Working quickly add the melted chocolate, cacao and vanilla.

6: Gently '*fold*' in the whisked egg white mixture using a spatula in 1/3 even batches, fold softly making sure not to deflate.

7: Once you have mixed the batter together pour into your prepared buttered and floured ramekins. Place in the oven at 190'c for approximately 10-12 mins depending on your oven. Do not open the door during the cooking process. You will start to see the souffle rise.

8: Dust with the sugar free icing and serve immediately.

Nutrition Facts

Amount per
1 serving (2.2 oz) — 63 g

Calories 135	From Fat	103
	% Daily Value*	
Total Fat 11.6g		18%
Saturated Fat 6.4g		32%
Trans Fat 0g		
Cholesterol 234mg		78%
Sodium 173mg		7%
Total Carbohydrates 7g		2%
Dietary Fiber 1g		4%
Sugars 0g		
Protein 4g		9%
Vitamin A 7%	Vitamin C	0%
Calcium 3%	Iron	7%

* Percent Daily Values are based on 2000 calorie diet. Your Daily Values may be higher or lower depending on your calorie needs.

HappyForks.com

Chocolate Panna Cotta

Yield: Serves 8-10

Ingredients

400g   Sugar-free dark chocolate
2 ½ cups Coconut milk
4 Tbsp Stevia
I tsps. Vanilla extract
2 ½ Tbsp Powdered gelatin,
(*dissolved in 2 cups of boiling water*)

Optional:
Berries, oranges or roasted hazelnut;
coconut cream or
natural yoghurt to serve

DIRECTIONS

1: In a pan over medium heat, heat milk until it begins to simmer.

2: chocolate, stevia and vanilla extract and stir gently with a whisk for a few minutes until mixture reaches boiling point.

3: Add the gelatin mixture (through a strainer to avoid any lumps forming) to the chocolate and continue to whisk overheat until well combined.

4: Remove from heat and pour into individual silicon molds. Allow to cool slightly before placing in the fridge to chill and set for several hours or overnight.

5: Turn out from molds and serve with fresh orange segments or berries, crushed roasted hazelnuts and a dollop of whipped coconut cream or natural yoghurt.

<u>Hint:</u> A spoonful of grated sugar-free dark chocolate also goes deliciously well on top.

Nutrition Facts
Amount per 103 g
1 serving (3.6 oz)
Calories 162
From fat 127
HappyForks.com

	Amount	% Daily Value*		Amount	% Daily Value*
Total Fat	15.1g	23%	Total Carbohydrates	9g	3%
Saturated	13g	65%	Dietary Fiber	3g	10%
Trans Fat	0g		Sugars	2g	
Cholesterol	0mg	0%	Protein	4g	8%
Sodium	150mg	6%			
Calcium	1%	Iron 10%	Vitamin A	0%	Vitamin C 3%

* Percent Daily Values are based on 2000 calorie diet. Your Daily Values may be higher or lower depending on your calorie needs

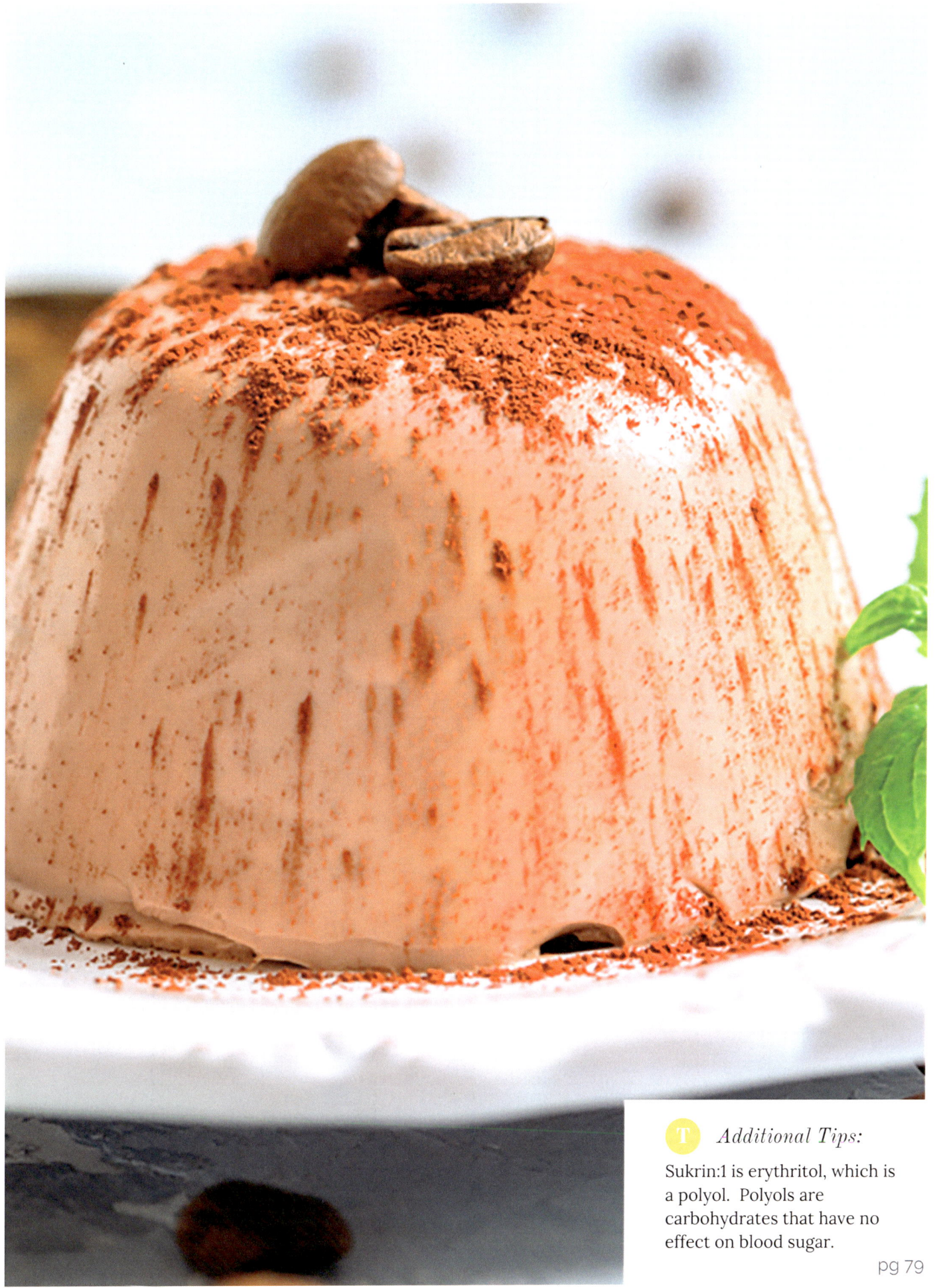

Additional Tips:

Sukrin:1 is erythritol, which is a polyol. Polyols are carbohydrates that have no effect on blood sugar.

Steamed Chocolate Orange Pudding with Chocolate Custard

Yield: Serves - 4 puddings

Ingredients

Pudding
100g Butter
100g Almond Flour
1 tsps. Baking powder (gluten free)
100g Powdered stevia
2 Eggs
25g Cocoa powder – *sifted*
Zest of 2 oranges
25g Sugar free dark chocolate

Chocolate Custard
2 Egg yolks
1 Tbsp Powdered stevia
1 Tbsp rice flour
300ml Coconut milk
100g Sugar-free dark chocolate

DIRECTIONS

1: Lightly grease 4 individual pudding basins.

2: Place butter and sugar in a bowl and mix until light and fluffy.

3: Add one egg at a time mixing well

4: Chop the chocolate and zest 2 oranges and stir into the mixture.

5: Add sifted cocoa and flour and mix until combined.

6: Spoon the mixture into the prepared basins and level the tops. . The mixture should fill the basins.

7: Cover puddings with a piece of foil wrap and using a rubber secure to the pudding basins.

8: Steam for 45 minutes, until puddings are cooked and springy to the touch.

Make the custard

1: To make the custard beat, together egg yolks, sugar and rice flour to form a smooth paste.

2: Remove from the heat, add the chocolate and stir until the chocolate melts.

3: Lift the puddings from the steamer, run a knife around the edges of the basins and turn out on to a serving plates.

4: Drizzle chocolate custard over and serve with extra thinly sliced ginger.

Nutrition Facts

Amount per 1 serving (7.8 oz): 222 g
Calories: 562
From fat: 352

Amount	% Daily Value*	Amount	% Daily Value*
Total Fat 40g	61%	Total Carbohydrates 38g	13%
Saturated 14.8g	74%	Dietary Fiber 9g	36%
Trans Fat 0g		Sugars 18g	
Cholesterol 442mg	147%	Protein 21g	42%
Sodium 398mg	17%		
Calcium 26% • Iron 31%		Vitamin A 104% • Vitamin C 50%	

*Percent Daily Values are based on 2000 calorie diet. Your Daily Values may be

HappyForks.com

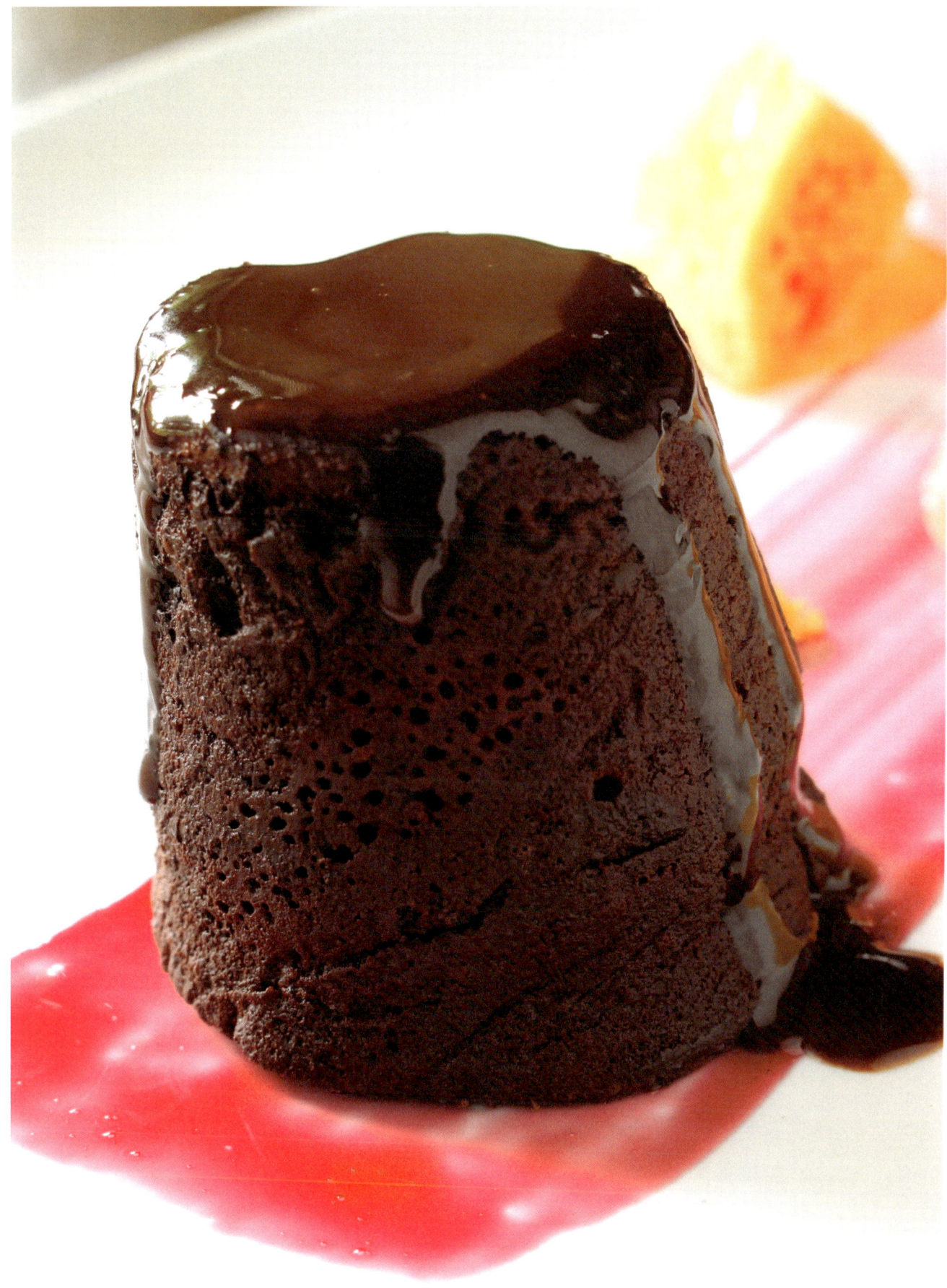

pg 81

Dairy Free - Chocolate Mousse

The tip to get a really thick mousse is to leave the can of coconut cream in the fridge before opening the can. Then spoon out the hardened cream that has risen to the top.

Serves 12

Ingredients

1 Tbsp Organic cocoa powder
300ml Organic coconut cream
2 Tbsp Stevia liquid drops

DIRECTIONS

1: Place your coconut cream in the fridge – preferably overnight. This will allow the cream to separate from the coconut water.

2: In a small container place the cocoa powder and add very small amount of hot water to make a paste. Stir to remove the lumps.

3: Add the stevia to the cocoa and combine.

4: Remove the coconut cream from the fridge – open the can and scoop out the cream – it should have come to surface and separated from the coconut water. Scoop out all the cream until you get to the water. You can keep this for using in smoothies etc.

5: Add the cocoa/stevia paste to the coconut cream and whisk to combine.

6: Spoon into jars – enjoy straight away or chill and serve.

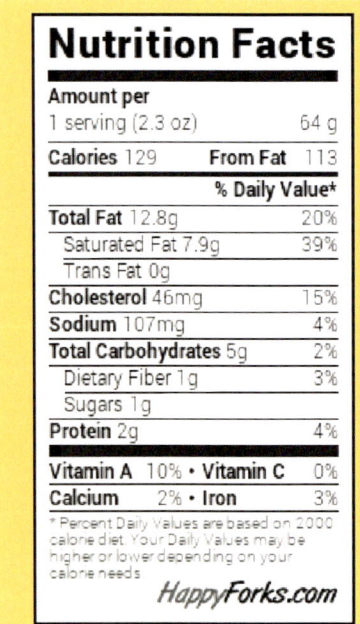

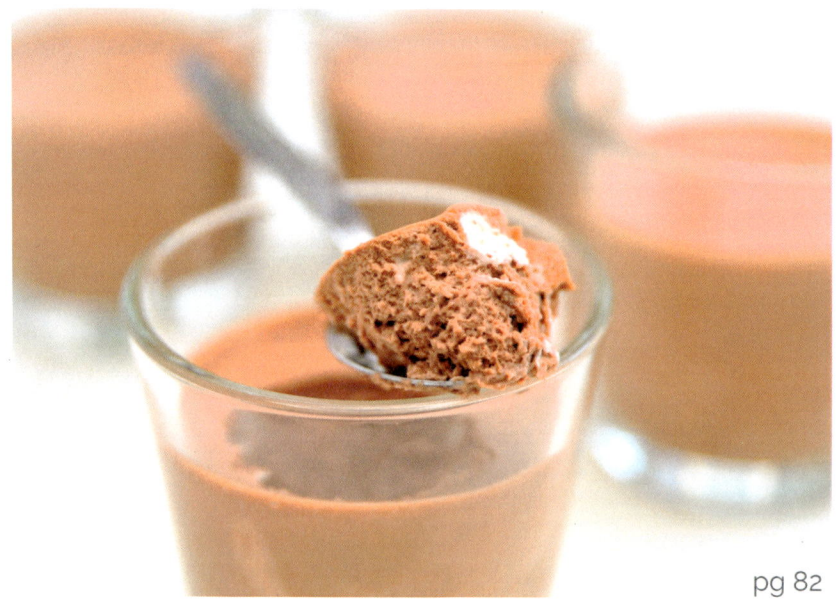

Chocolate Truffle Cr'eme Brulee`

The classic creme brulee is a dinner favourite but this sugar free chocolate one will be a dinner party success that you can make in advance to reduce the stress.

Yield : Makes 4 Ramekins

Ingredients

2 cups heavy cream
5 large egg yolks
⅓ cup Powdered stevia
½ tsp Liquid Stevia
100g Sugar free dark chocolate
optional 2 tbsp Brandy essence

Optional Toppings
Sugar Free icing sugar(sukrin)
whipped cream
Grated Sugar free dark chocolate

DIRECTIONS

1: Preparation: Preheat oven to 160 degrees and place rack to the middle position. Heat water in a kettle until hot, not boiling. Find a pan large enough to fit the 4 ramekins, whilst deep enough to add water half way up the sides of the ramekins.

2: Chop the chocolate into slivers.

3: Add the yolks and 1 tbsp of the Powdered sweetener to a medium bowl. Beat well to completely break up the yolks.

4: Pour the heavy cream into a small saucepan and add the remaining granulated sweetener, and Liquid stevia. Place on a medium heat, stirring occasionally with a whisk, until bubbles begin to simmer around the edge of the mixture. Turn off the heat and begin pouring the egg yolk into the hot cream mixture - very slowly in a thin stream, while quickly whisking all the while. Add the chopped chocolate and stir to melt and combine. Whisk in the brandy.

5: Divide the chocolate truffle creme brulee mixture evenly between 4 ramekins. Place the ramekins into the pan and fill the pan with hot water half way up the sides of the ramekins. Carefully place the pan into the oven and bake for 30 minutes or until the very center of the creme brulee is barely wobbling.

6: Cool the chocolate truffle creme brulee in the water bath for an hour before removing to a rack to cool completely. Cover with plastic wrap and refrigerate at least 4 hours but overnight is better.

7: Before serving, sprinkle 1/2 teaspoon sugar free icing over the top of each creme brulee. Melt the sweetener with a culinary torch until it caramelizes, turning brown. Alternately, add a dollop of whipped cream to the top. Serve.

Nutrition Facts

Amount per 1 serving (4 oz) — 115 g

Calories 304 — From Fat 260

	% Daily Value*
Total Fat 29.4g	45%
Saturated Fat 16.7g	84%
Trans Fat 0g	
Cholesterol 313mg	104%
Sodium 120mg	5%
Total Carbohydrates 10g	3%
Dietary Fiber 3g	12%
Sugars 2g	
Protein 7g	13%
Vitamin A 24% • Vitamin C	1%
Calcium 7% • Iron	12%

* Percent Daily Values are based on 2000 calorie diet. Your Daily Values may be higher or lower depending on your calorie needs

HappyForks.com

Sacher Torte

Ingredients:

Cake
150g   Sugar-free dark chocolate
½ cup   Butter (*at room temperature*)
¾ cup   Stevia (*powdered*)
6 Large eggs (*separated and at room temperature*)
1 tsps. Vanilla extract
½ cup Stevia sweetener (*powdered*) (*this will be added with the egg white*)
1 cup   Almond flour (*sifted to remove any clumps*)

Filling
⅓ cup   Sugar-free apricot jam
2 Tbsp   Water

Chocolate Glaze
¾ cup Whipping cream
⅓ cup   Powdered stevia
100g Sugar-free dark chocolate
½ tsps. Vanilla extract

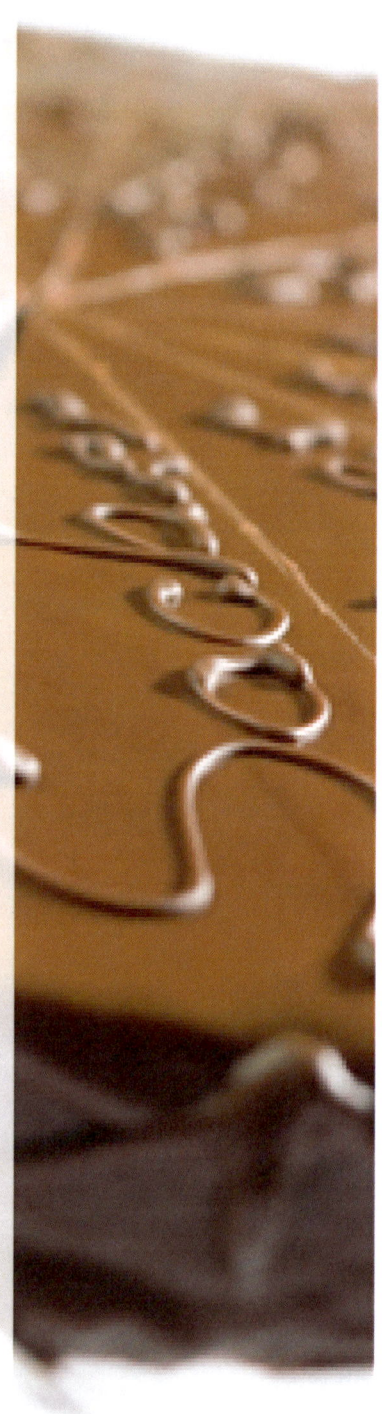

Sacher Torte

Method

1. Preheat oven to 160 Degrees and grease a 9-inch springform pan. Line the bottom with baking paper.

2. In a small saucepan over low heat, melt the chocolate until smooth. Set aside to cool.

3. In a large bowl, beat butter until smooth. Beat in powdered sweetener for several minutes until well combined and smooth. Beat in egg yolks, one at a time, scraping down sides of bowl and beaters as needed. Add chocolate and vanilla extract and beat until well combined.

4. In another large bowl, beat the egg whites until frothy. Add granulated sweetener and beat on high until soft peaks form. Stir about one third of the whites into the chocolate mixture to lighten it, then fold in the remaining whites being careful to not deflate.

5. Add sifted almond flour and fold in until just combined. Spread batter in prepared pan and bake 30 to 40 minutes, or until set and a skewer inserted in the centre comes out clean. Remove and let cool completely.

6. Run a sharp knife around the edges of the pan to loosen and then remove pan sides. Flip cake out onto a wire rack and carefully cut into two horizontal layers. Carefully transfer one layer to a serving platter (use two large flipping spatulas to help you move the layer without cracking).

7. In a small bowl, whisk together the apricot jam and water until well combined. Spread about 2/3 of the filling over the first layer of cake. Carefully top with the second layer of cake and spread with remaining filling. Refrigerate while preparing the glaze.

8. In a small saucepan over medium heat, whisk together whipping cream and powdered sweetener. Bring to just a simmer, then remove from heat and add chopped chocolate and vanilla. Let sit 5 minutes to melt and then whisk until smooth. Let cool 10 minutes to thicken.

9. Pour glaze over the top of the cake, spreading to the edges. Let it drip slowly down the sides, spreading all over to cover completely.

10. Refrigerate until glaze is set, about 1 hour. To cut into slices, warm a sharp knife in hot water.
Serve with whipped cream.

Nutrition Facts

Amount per 1 serving (2.5 oz): 70 g
Calories: 184
From fat: 105

Amount	% Daily Value*	Amount	% Daily Value*
Total Fat 11.9g	18%	Total Carbohydrates 19g	6%
Saturated 6.7g	33%	Dietary Fiber 0g	1%
Trans Fat 0g		Sugars 15g	
Cholesterol 117mg	39%	Protein 2g	4%
Sodium 44mg	2%		
Calcium 2% • Iron 2%		Vitamin A 9% • Vitamin C 12%	

* Percent Daily Values are based on a 2000 calorie diet. Your Daily Values may be higher or lower depending on your calorie needs.

HappyForks.com

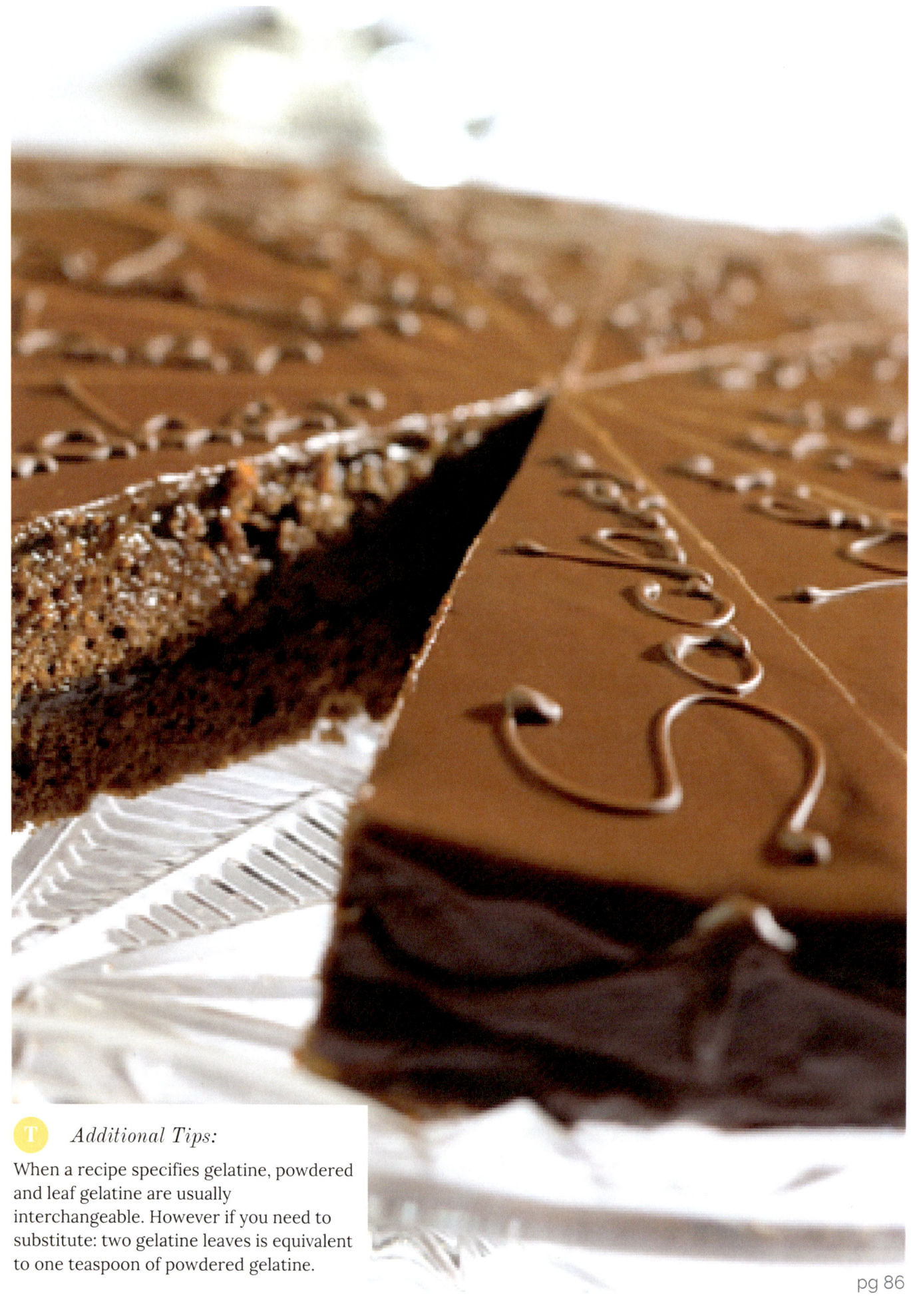

T *Additional Tips:*

When a recipe specifies gelatine, powdered and leaf gelatine are usually interchangeable. However if you need to substitute: two gelatine leaves is equivalent to one teaspoon of powdered gelatine.

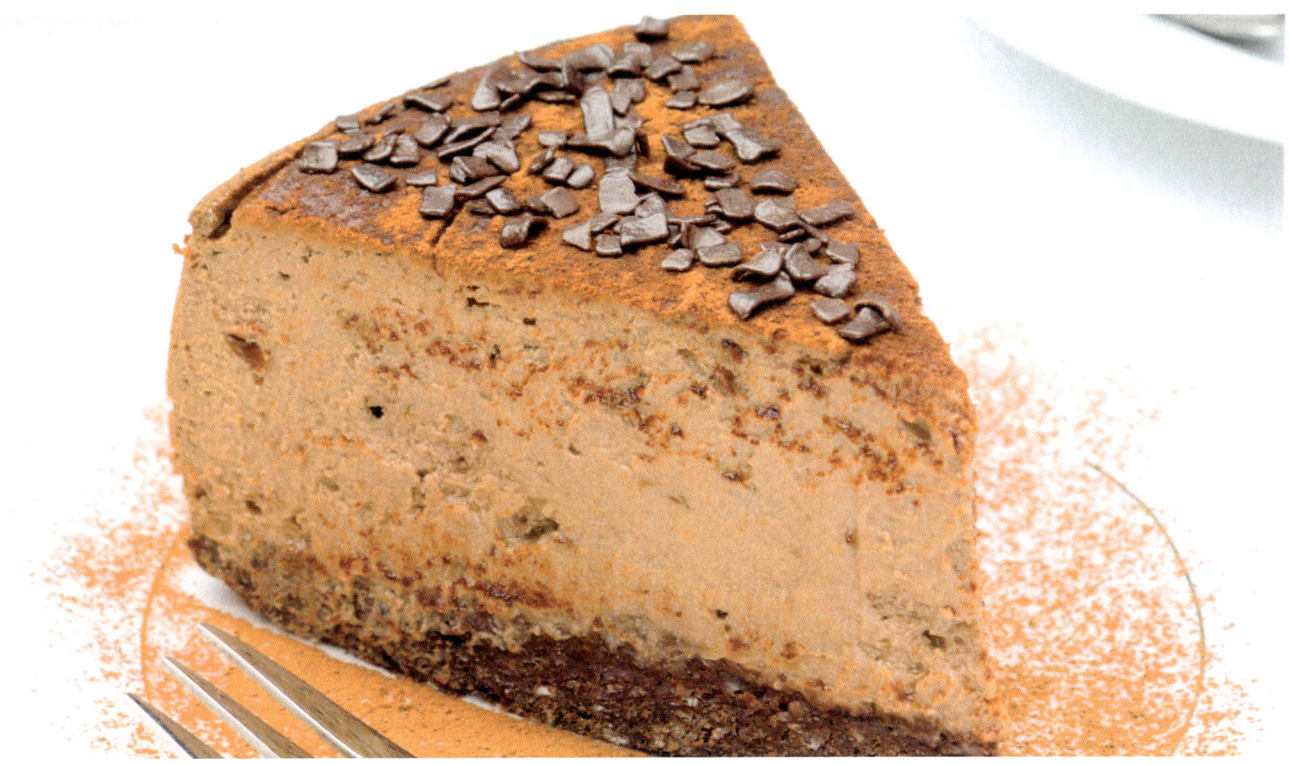

Baked Chocolate Cheesecake

Ingredients

Cake
- 180g Sugar free dark chocolate
- 500g cream cheese (*at room temperature*)
- 4 Eggs
- 2 Tbsp Cacao powder
- 1 cup Greek yoghurt
- 1 Tbsp powdered Stevia

Base
- 250g Roasted Almonds
- 100g Walnut Kernels
- 250g Melted Butter

Frosting (optional)
- 8 Tbsp Smooth, natural peanut butter
- 200g Cream cheese, (*at room temperature*)
- ½ tsps. Salt
- ½ tsps. Stevia
- 6 Tbsp Coconut milk

Nutrition Facts

Amount per 1 serving (6.5 oz): 185 g
Calories 584, From fat 455

Amount	% Daily Value*	Amount	% Daily Value*
Total Fat 51.9g	80%	Total Carbohydrates 17g	6%
Saturated 20.8g	104%	Dietary Fiber 4g	18%
Trans Fat 0g		Sugars 6g	
Cholesterol 282mg	94%	Protein 19g	38%
Sodium 606mg	25%		
Calcium 17% • Iron 19%		Vitamin A 23% • Vitamin C 1%	

*Percent Daily Values are based on 2000 calorie diet. Your Daily Values may be higher or lower depending on your calorie needs.

HappyForks.com

Baked Chocolate Cheesecake

DIRECTIONS

1. Pre-heat oven to 160°C and line a 25cm cake tin with baking paper.

2. To make the base, use a food processor to turn the almonds and walnuts into a breadcrumb-like consistency.

3. Add the melted butter and combine well.

4. Spoon the mixture into your prepared tin and spread evenly over the base, using a dessert spoon or your hands.

5. Place in the fridge to set while you prepare the filling.

6. To make the filling, use electric beaters or a mixer to combine the cream cheese and eggs.

7. Once smooth, stir through the yoghurt, cacao powder and stevia.

8. Melt dark chocolate (either over a double-boiler or broken up in the microwave on high in 30 second batches, stirring in between) and, while hot, pour into the cream cheese mixture a little at a time, stirring in between to make sure it combines before setting.

9. Remove the base from the fridge and pour in the filling. Tap the cake tin lightly on the bench to remove any air bubbles.

10. Bake at 160°C for 60-75 minutes, or until the middle of the cake has set by testing a skewer comes out clean. Once cooked, turn off the oven and leave the cake in with the door ajar (*this prevents any cracks forming on the top of the cake from rapid temperature changes.*)

11. Once cooled, place the cake in the fridge.

12. To prepare the peanut butter frosting, use an electric mixer to whip together the cream cheese, peanut butter, salt, stevia and milk. If the mixture feels too firm to pipe, add a little extra milk one tablespoon at a time (it will depend on the brand of peanut butter you buy).

13. Spread the peanut butter frosting into the cake (or just it evenly if you prefer).

14. Serve the cake chilled with fresh extra cream.

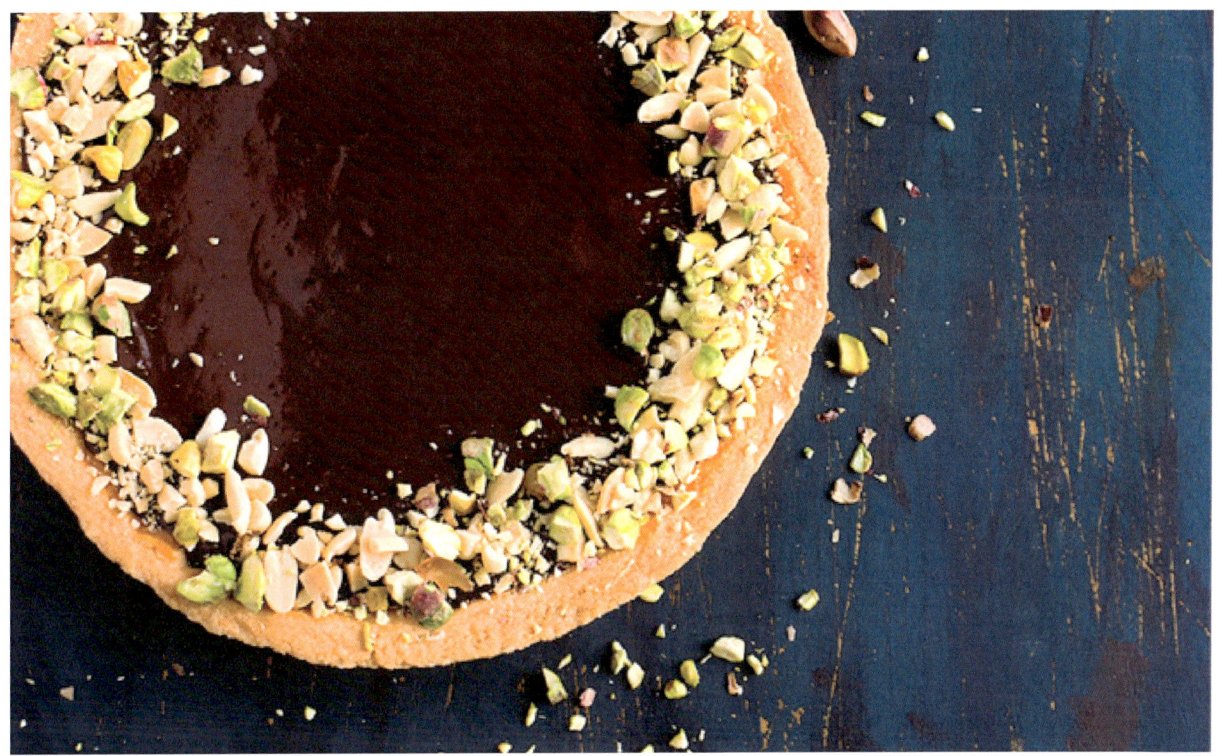

Ganache Tart with Crunchy Macadamia, Pistachio and Coconut Topping

Ingredients

Yield: Makes 1 large cake, 12 slices

Tart base
- 1 ½ cups Fine almond meal
- ¼ tsps. Himalayan salt
- 2 Tbsp Stevia
- ½ cup Unsweetened shredded coconut
- 2 tablespoons Extra virgin organic Coconut oil, melted
- 1 Egg

Ganache:
- 200g Sugar-free dark chocolate
- 1 cup Coconut cream
- 1 tsps. Vanilla extract

Topping:
- ⅓ cup Unsweetened coconut flakes
- ½ cup Raw macadamia nuts, (coarsely chopped)
- ½ cup Raw Pistachio nuts coarsely chopped)

Nutrition Facts
Amount per 128 g
1 serving (4.5 oz)
Calories 317
From fat 260
HappyForks.com

Amount	% Daily Value*	Amount	% Daily Value*
Total Fat 30.7g	47%	Total Carbohydrates 14g	5%
Saturated 16.3g	82%	Dietary Fiber 4g	14%
Trans Fat 0g		Sugars 3g	
Cholesterol 103mg	34%	Protein 5g	10%
Sodium 265mg	11%		
Calcium 3% • Iron 14%		Vitamin A 2% • Vitamin C 3%

*Percent Daily Values are based on 2000 calorie diet. Your Daily Values may be higher or lower depending on your calorie needs.

Ganache Tart with Crunchy Macadamia, Pistachio and Coconut Topping

DIRECTIONS

1. Preheat oven to 180°C.

2. In a food processor, combine the almond meal, salt, stevia and shredded coconut until it resembles a fine crumb.

3. Add the melted coconut oil and egg to the almond meal and coconut mixture. Blend until coarse crumbs form and when squeezed between fingers, should form a dough.

4. Transfer dough to an 8-inch, greased flan tin with removable bottom, and using a flat-bottomed glass or your fingers, press dough evenly into the bottom and up the sides of the tin – ensuring it's of even thickness.

5. Bake in oven until golden and cooked through, approximately 18-20 minutes, then transfer to a wire rack to cool completely.

6. Spread the chopped macadamia nuts, pistachios and shredded coconut evenly onto a baking paper-lined tray and bake until lightly golden. Be sure to keep an eye on it to ensure it doesn't burn. Set aside to cool.

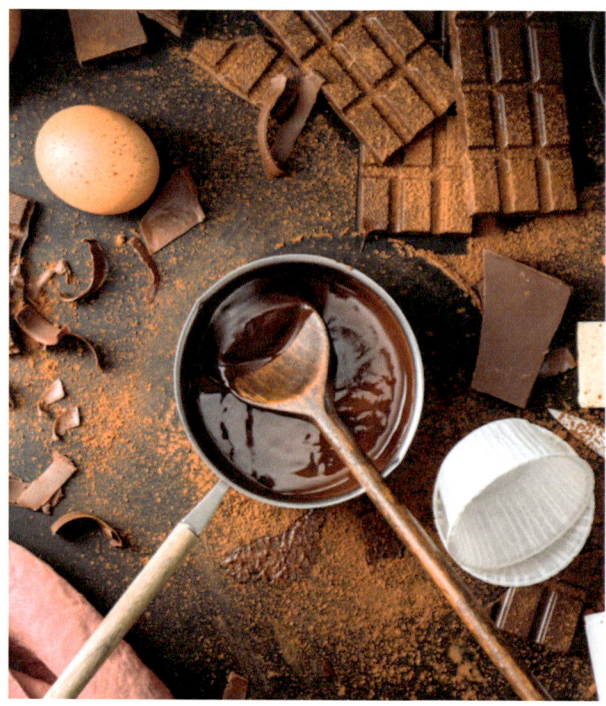

7. To make the ganache, place sugar-free dark chocolate in a large mixing bowl, and in a separate small saucepan, bring coconut cream to a simmer. Pour hot coconut cream over the chocolate, sit for 30 seconds, and then stir until smooth and creamy before mixing in the vanilla extract.

8. To assemble the tart, pour chocolate ganache into cooled tart shell and scatter the toasted macadamias, pistachios and toasted coconut over the top. Sprinkle with some freshly grated nutmeg if desired and refrigerate for at least 1-2 hours or until set.

Tiramisu Swiss Roll

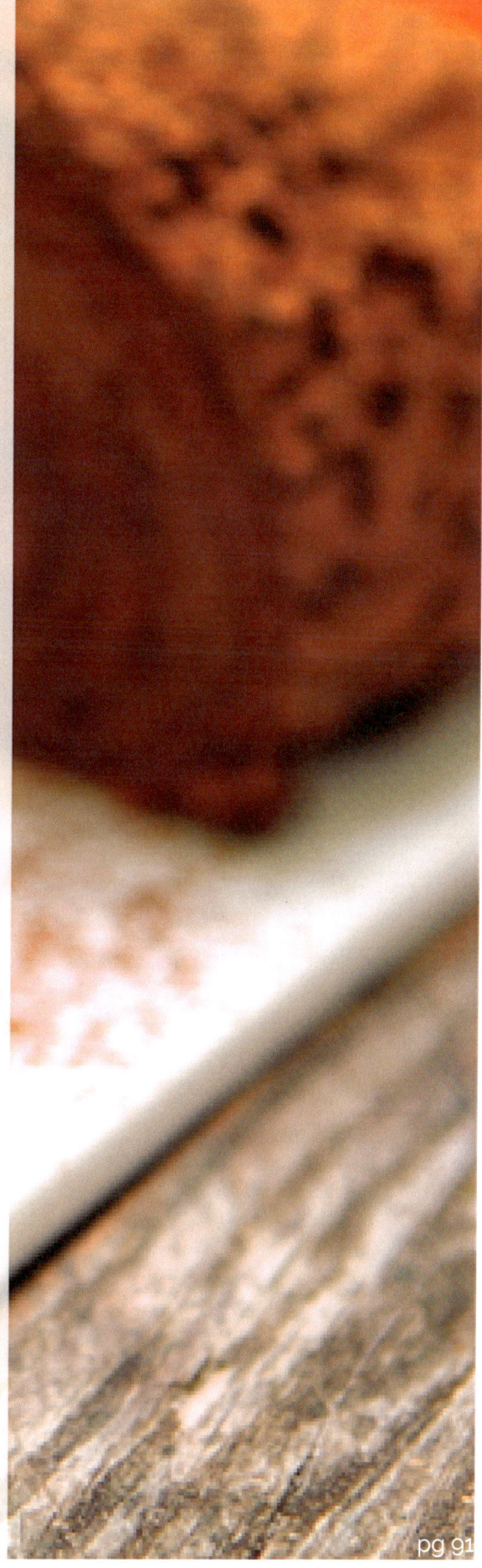

Ingredients:

Cake
30g Sugar free dark chocolate
⅓ cup Coconut flour
¼ cup Unsweetened cocoa powder
1 Tbsp Psyllium fiber powder
¼ tsps. Baking soda
¼ tsps. Salt
6 Eggs room temp
1 Tbsp Instant espresso
½ cup Powdered Stevia
1 tsps. Chocolate liquid stevia

Syrup
¼ cup Water
1 Tbsp Strong cooled coffee
½ tsps. Coffee extract
½ tsps. Chocolate liquid stevia

Filling
150g Mascarpone cheese
2 Tbsp Strong cooled coffee
2 Tbsp Unsweetened cocoa powder
½ tsps. Liquid stevia
½ tsps. Coffee extract
¼ cup Heavy whipping cream

Ganache
½ cup Heavy cream
¼ cup Unsweetened cocoa powder
½ tsps. Coffee extract
½ tsps. Liquid stevia

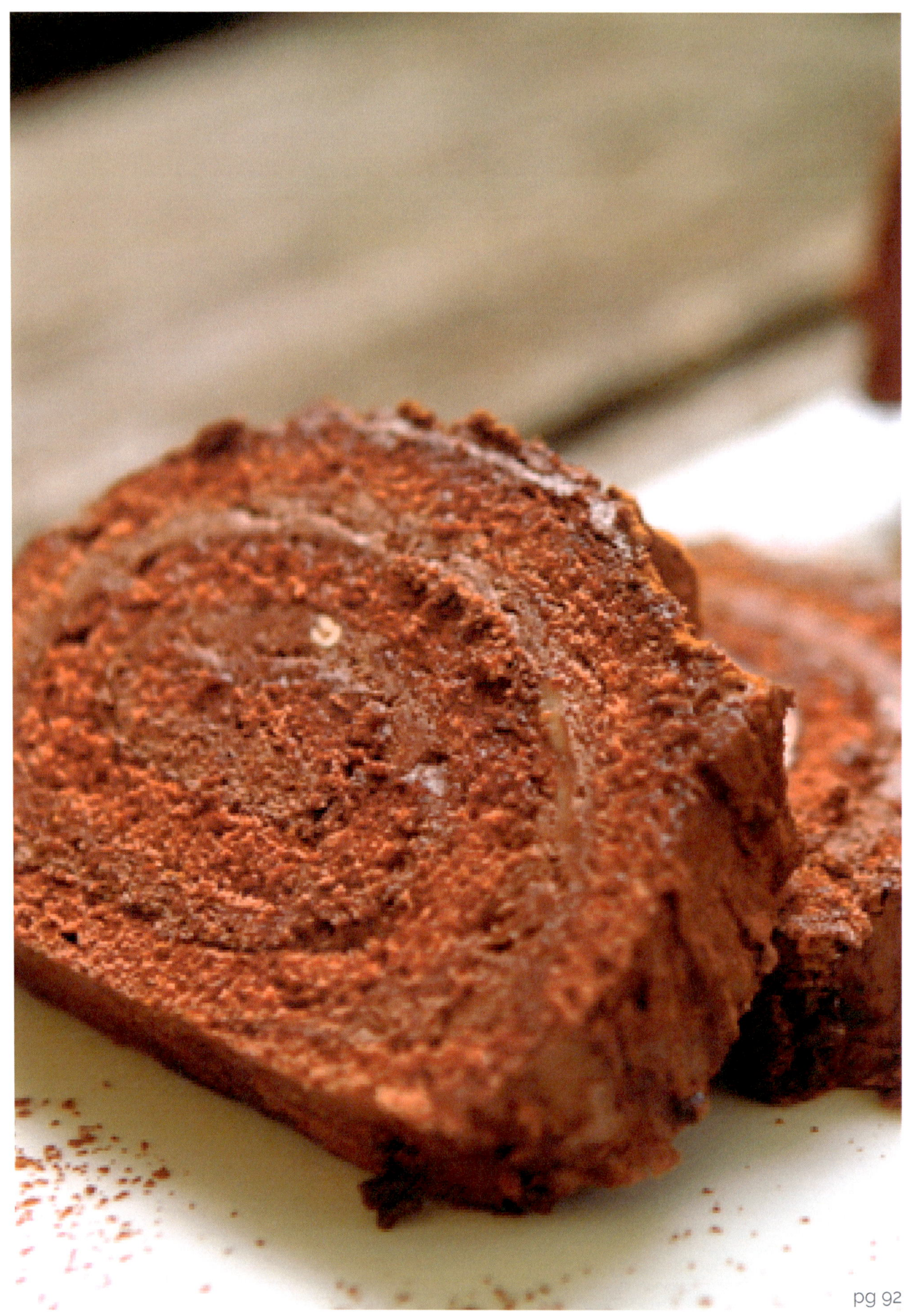

Chocolate Tiramisu Swiss Roll

Method

1. Preheat oven to 180 degrees Celsius.

2. Line a baking sheet with baking paper and grease. Set aside.

3. Chop the chocolate in a food processor until fine crumbs.

4. Add the remaining dry ingredients into the food processor and blend until combined.

5. In a mixer add the eggs and remaining ingredients for the cake and blend until combined.

6. Slowly pour in the dry ingredients into the wet mixture and blend until combined.

7. Spread this onto the baking pan.

8. Bake for approx. 10 minutes.

9. Remove immediately and sprinkle with a little unsweetened cocoa powder over the cake.

10. Cover with a clean linen tea-towel. Place another baking pan the same size and flip over.

11. Immediately and carefully remove the baking paper on this side. Sprinkle with more cocoa powder and another clean towel or use baking paper.

12. Roll up, starting at the short side, while the cake is still warm. Allow to cool completely.

13. Once cooled, unroll carefully.

14. Whisk together the syrup ingredients and use a pastry brush to cover the cake with the syrup.

15. Make the filling in a stand mixer, blend on high until smooth and spread evenly over the entire cake.

16. Roll cake up, cover with baking paper, and refrigerate for at least 2 hours.

To make the ganache:

1. Heat the cream in a saucepan over low heat, until just gently simmering, do not boil. Remove from heat and whisk in the remaining ingredients. Taste and adjust sweetener if needed.

2. Cover cake with ganache and refrigerate. Use baking paper over both rolled ends but leave the ganache on top uncovered in the fridge.

3. Allow to chill for 3 hours or overnight before serving.

Nutrition Facts
Amount per 1 serving (3 oz) 84 g
Calories 157
From fat 109

Amount	% Daily Value
Total Fat 12.3g	19%
Saturated 5.9g	29%
Trans Fat 0g	
Cholesterol 327mg	109%
Sodium 314mg	13%
Calcium 11% • Iron 14%	

Amount	% Daily Value
Total Carbohydrates 9g	3%
Dietary Fiber 2g	7%
Sugars 2g	
Protein 8g	16%
Vitamin A 9% • Vitamin C 0%	

*Percent Daily Values are based on a 2000 calorie diet. Your Daily Values may be higher or lower depending on your calorie needs.

HappyForks.com

Black Forrest Gateau

Technically cherries are not considered a strict ketogenic fruit being slightly higher in fructose than the more suitable berries family.
However when a special occasion calls - what better way to celebrate than a sugar-free version of a classic black forrest.

1 large cake serves 16

Ingredients

Cake

150g Sugar-free dark chocolate
½ cup Butter
(*at room temperature*)
¾ cup Stevia (*powdered*)
6 Large eggs
(*separated, room temperature*)
1 tsps. Vanilla extract
½ cup Stevia sweetener (*powdered*)
(*this will be added with the egg white*)
1 cup Almond flour
(*sifted to remove any clumps*)

Amarenta

375g pitted cherries
(*Frozen is fine*)
8 tsps. Liquid stevia
¾ cup water
2 tbsp Ground chia seeds

Filling:

1 *recipe Low-Carb *Amarenata*
720 ml heavy whipping cream
300g full-fat cream cheese

Garnishes

16-20 large fresh cherries
50g sugar-free chocolate(*grated*)

DIRECTIONS

1: Make the Amarenta first. Wash the cherries and remove the pits. Add them to a stainless steel pan.

2: Add the stevia, 3/4 cup of water and the 2 tablespoons of chia seed.

3: Place on a stove and cook over low-medium heat. Slowly bring to a boil and mix frequently until the juices slightly thicken. This may take 20-30 minutes. When done, your amarenata should be thickened into a syrup and the flavour very strong - just like sweet cherry extract. It will thicken even more when chilled.

4: You can store amarenata in the fridge for up to 2 weeks or preserve for longer. You will need 1/2 cups of this recipe for the cake layers to decorate the black forrest cake.

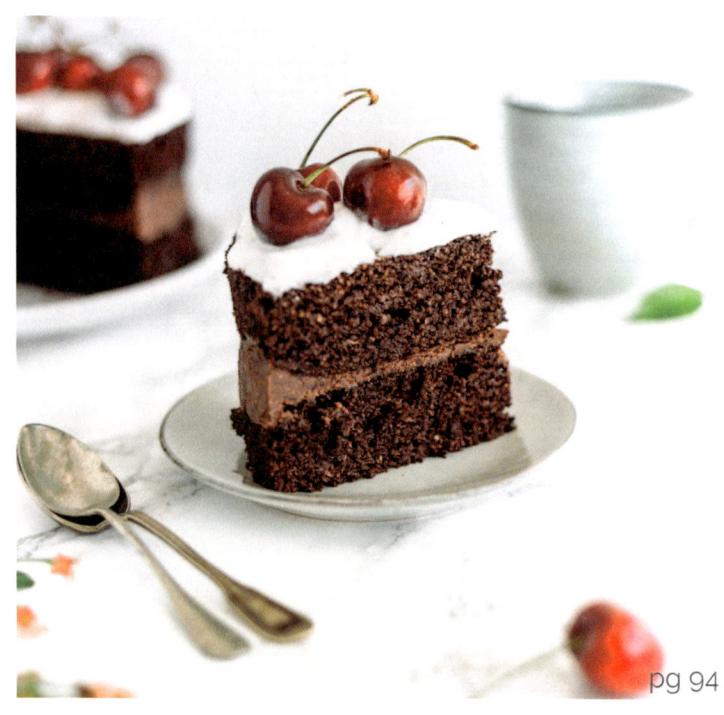

Black Forrest Gateau

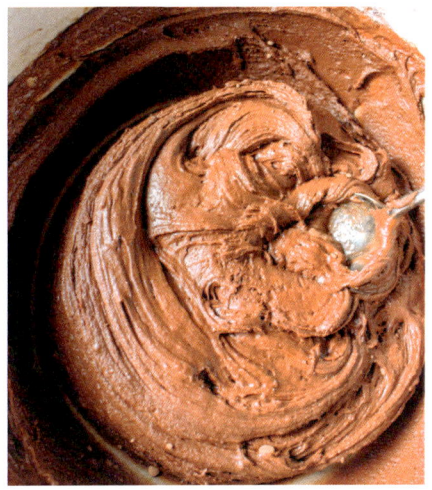
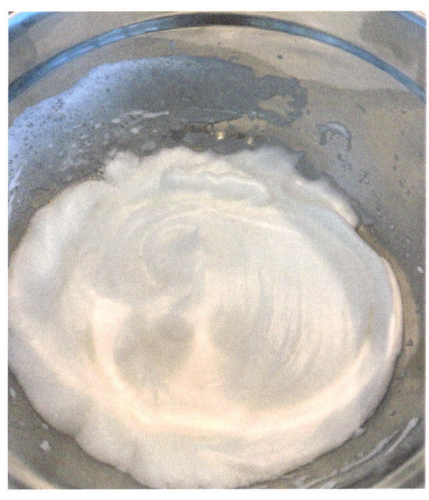
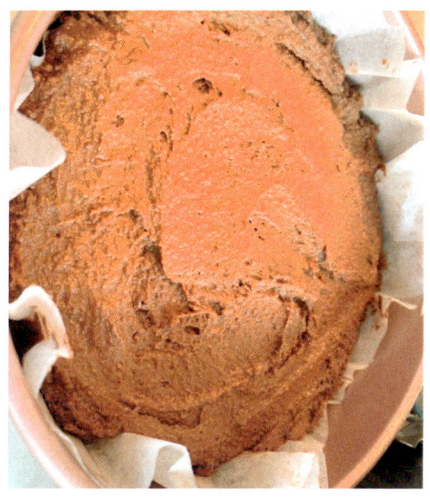

Step 1-3:

1 Pre-heat the oven to 160 °C. Grease 3 x 9-inch springform pan. Line the bottom with baking paper.

Note:
It is recommended you cook these in 3 separate pans rather than trying to cut one cake into 3 layers horizontally after cooking to prevent breaking.

2. In a small saucepan over low heat, melt the chocolate until smooth. Set aside to cool.

3. In a large bowl, beat butter until smooth. Beat in powdered sweetener for several minutes until well combined and smooth. Beat in egg yolks, one at a time, scraping down sides of bowl and beaters as needed. Add the melted chocolate and vanilla extract and beat until well combined.

Step 4:

4. In another large bowl, beat the egg whites until frothy. Add granulated sweetener and beat on high until soft peaks form.

 Stir about one third of the whites into the chocolate mixture to lighten it, then fold in the remaining whites being careful to not deflate.

Step 5-7:

5. Add sifted almond flour and fold in until just combined. Spread batter in prepared pan and bake 30 to 40 minutes, or until set and a skewer inserted in the centre comes out clean. Remove and let cool completely.

6. Run a sharp knife around the edges of the pan to loosen and then remove pan sides. Flip cake out onto a wire rack

7. Allow the cake to completely cool prior to the assembly stage.

Black Forrest Gateau-Assembly

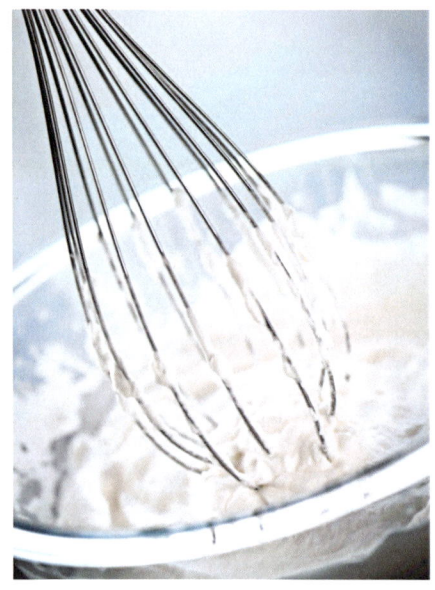
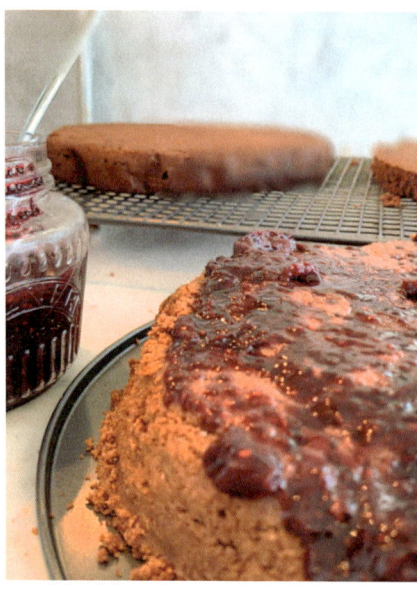
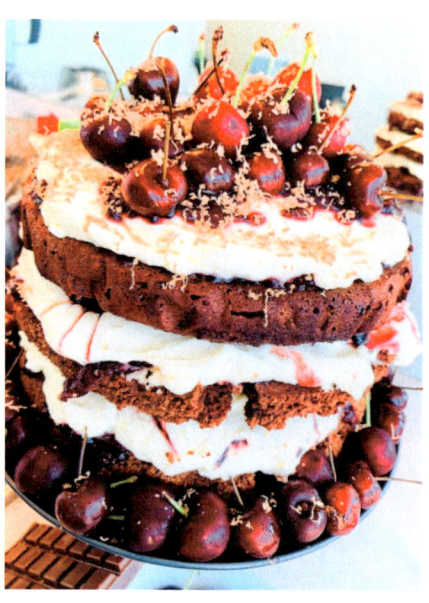

Step 1-2:

1. To make the filling, in a bowl beat the cream and cream cheese.
Optionally, add sweetener to taste.

2. Start assembling the cake (note: you have 3 chocolate cake layers, and you will need to divide the amarenata into 3 parts and the cream into 3 parts). Place the first cake layer, cut side up, on a cake tray. Spread about 2 tablespoons of the Amarenata syrup (without cherry pieces) on top and let it soak in. Add about a third of the mascarpone-cream topping.

Step 3-5:

3. Top with about a third of the Amarenata.

4. Add the second cake layer and repeat the process: top with about 2 tablespoons of the Amarenata syrup, a third of the cream and a third of the Amarenata.

5. Top with the third and last cake layer. Add the remaining Amarenata and let the syrup soak in.

Step 6-7:

6. Spread the-cream layer on top. Optionally, decorate with fresh cherries and grated sugar free chocolate. Refrigerate for at least 2 hours to set before slicing.

7. Slice and serve!

Nutrition Facts

Amount per
1 serving (5.5 oz) — 156 g

Calories 287 — From Fat 231

% Daily Value*

Total Fat 26.1g	40%
Saturated Fat 15.6g	78%
Trans Fat 0g	
Cholesterol 150mg	50%
Sodium 255mg	11%
Total Carbohydrates 25g	8%
Dietary Fiber 1g	4%
Sugars 6g	
Protein 6g	12%

Vitamin A 20% • Vitamin C 6%
Calcium 9% • Iron 4%

Handy Conversion Chart

VOLUME (DRY)

1/8 teaspoon	0.5 ml
1/4 teaspoon	1 ml
1/2 teaspoon	2 ml
3/4 teaspoon	4 ml
1 teaspoon	5 ml
1 tablespoon	15 ml
1/4 cup	59 ml
1/3 cup	79 ml
1/2 cup	118 ml
2/3 cup	158 ml
3/4 cup	177 ml
1 cup	225 ml
4 cups or 1 quart	1 liter

Handy Conversion Chart

WEIGHT (MASS)

American Standard (Ounces)	Metric (Grams)
1/2 ounce	14 grams
1 ounce	28 grams
3 ounces	85 grams
3.53 ounces	100 grams
4 ounces	113 grams
8 ounces	227 grams
12 ounces	340 grams
16 ounces or 1 pound	454 grams
2.2 pound	1 Kg

Handy Conversion Chart

VOLUME (LIQUID)

American Standard (Cups & Quarts)	American Standard (Ounces)	Metric (Milliliters & Liters)
2 tbsp	1 fl. oz.	30 ml
1/4 cup	2 fl. oz.	60 ml
1/2 cup	4 fl. oz.	125 ml
1 cup	8 fl. oz.	250 ml
1 1/2 cups	12 fl. oz.	375 ml
2 cups or 1 pint	16 fl. oz	500 ml
4 cups or 1 quart	32 fl. oz.	1000 ml or 1 liter
1 gallon	128 fl. oz.	4 liters

Handy Conversion Chart

OVEN TEMPERATURES

American Standard	Metric
250° F	130° C
300° F	150° C
350° F	180° C
400° F	200° C
450° F	230° C

Handy Conversion Chart

DRY MEASURE EQUIVALENTS

Spoons	Cups	Ounces	Grams
3 teaspoons	1 tablespoon	1/2 ounce	14.3 grams
2 tablespoons	1/8 cup	1/8 cup	28.3 grams
4 tablespoons	1/4 cup	2 ounces	56.7 grams
5 & 1/3 tablespoons	1/3 cup	2.6 ounces	75.6 grams
8 tablespoons	1/2 cup	4 ounces	113 grams
12 tablespoons	3/4 cup	6 ounces	0.375 pound
32 tablespoons	2 cups	16 ounces	1 pound

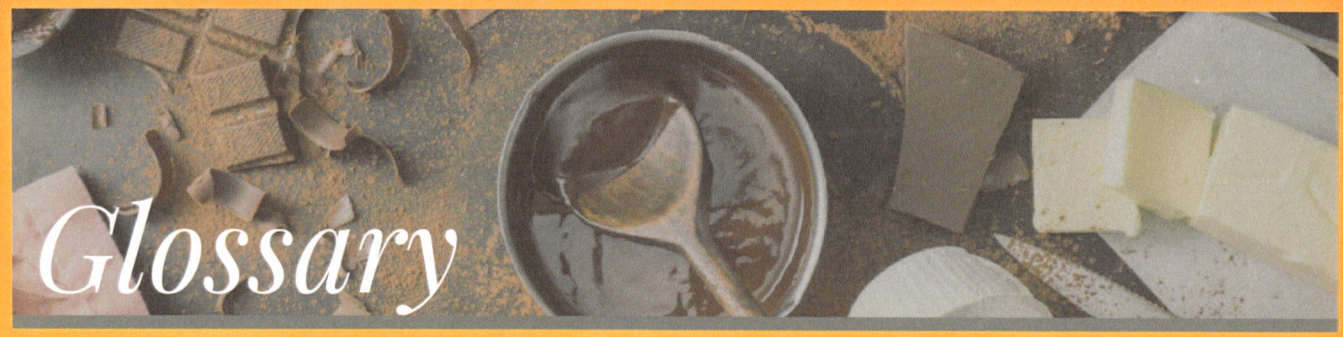

Glossary

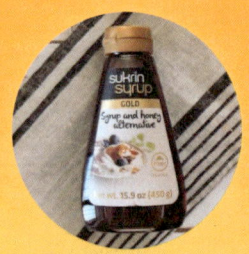

Sukrin sugar free syrup

low on calories and completely gluten-free. The low sugar content makes Syrup Gold very gentle on your blood sugar, and additionally, the syrup is both tooth-friendly and prebiotic.
Less than 1g of sugar 20g of dietary fiber 6g of sugar alcohol (erythritol) 2 net carbs

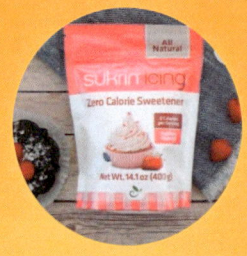

Sukrin sugar free icing sugar

A natural origin zero calorie alternative to regular powdered icing sugar. No artificial colours, additives or preservatives

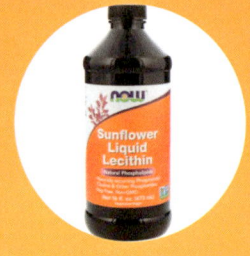

Sunflower-Liquid-Lecithin

Sunflower lecithin is rich in choline and other essential fatty acids such as phosphatidylinosito. Lecithin is essential in chocolate making as it aids in emulsifying fats, enabling them to be dispersed in water based liquids.

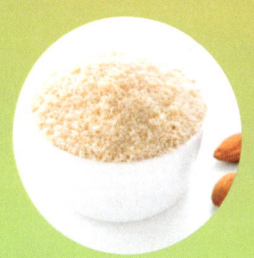

Almond flour

While almond meal is typically made from raw (unpeeled) almonds, almond flour is made from blanched (peeled) almonds. Compared to almond meal, almond flour has a finer texture and lighter color.

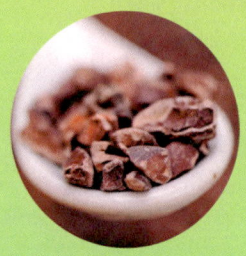

Cocoa nibs

Natural and organic with no added sweeteners or preservatives, they are simply crushed cacao beans.

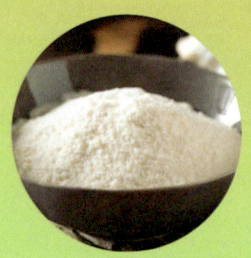

Coconut flour

Coconut flour is a soft, naturally grain- and gluten-free flour produced from dried coconut meat

References

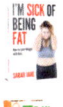

Contents of this book written by the author Sarah Jane.
Introduction chapters referenced from authors previous book:
- Sarah Jane .2018. **"I am sick of being fat** - "*How to lose weight with keto.*"

References to previous book by the author:
- Sarah Jane ,2020, "*7 day keto kick-starter*"

NAME OF CHAPTER:
Is a Ketogenic Diet Harmful or Dangerous?

http://diabetes.diabetesjournals.org/content/diabetes/suppl/2009/08/18/db08-1261.DC1/db08-1261_Online_appendix.pdf

IMAGES:
- Personal photographs of the author: Sarah Jane
- Other images purchased/licenced from Shutterstock/getty images
- Other images purchased/licenced Canva

ACKNOWLEDGEMENTS

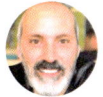

BOOK & RECIPE EDITING:
Very special thanks to Chef Pasqualino Candiloro

NUTRITIONAL LABELS
Created via online tool: https://www.happyforks.com recipe analyser.

WHERE TO SOURCE SPECIFIC INGREDIENTS:

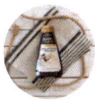

Recipes that require:
- sugar-free clear fibre syrup
- sugar-free gold fibre syrup
- sugar free icing sugar

can be obtained from this exclusive Australian supplier.

Click on this link to access : **http://sukrin.com.au/?aff=35**

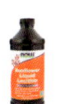

From recipe: "*No sugar white chocolate*"
click on this link:
https://www.amazon.com/NOW-Sunflower-Liquid-Lecithin-16-Ounce/dp/B00J8ET8IO?tag=wholyum-20

Full disclosure: Any affiliate commission that may be earned from the purchase of the products from these links are placed towards the cost of creating more educational material to help the health of many.

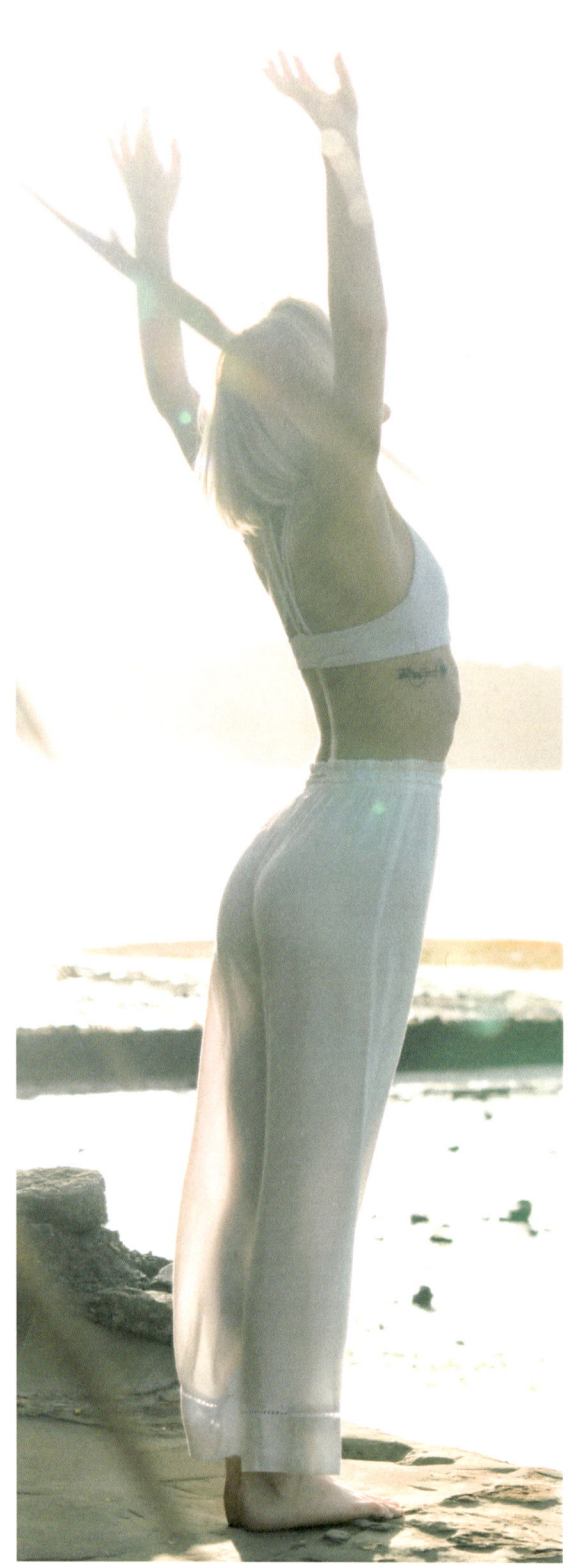

Thank You

It's been an absolute privilege and honour to share this information and recipes with you.

It is my hope that this cook-book has been a valuable resource for you.

It is my hope that you have learnt some science behind the success of a ketogenic diet.

It is my hope that you can see that a ketogenic diet doesn't mean depriving yourself of the sweet treats and enjoying the celebrations that life offers.

It is my hope that this has now propelled you to keep going.

So where to, now.....

If you have gained value from this book - then I invite you try my :

7 day keto challenge.
(www.7daychallenge.com.au)

Or if you ready to dive straight in:

- join the **30 day keto program**
"hormonal re-set"

Sarah Jane

www.ingramcontent.com/pod-product-compliance
Lightning Source LLC
Chambersburg PA
CBRC092339290426
44109CB00008B/166